Ophthalmic Ultrasound

To my wife and parents

For Churchill Livingstone

Commissioning Editor Geoff Nuttall
Copy Editor Colin Nicholls
Project Controllers Kay Hunston, Debra Barrie
Design Direction Erik Bigland

Ophthalmic Ultrasound

A PRACTICAL GUIDE

Hatem R. Atta FRCS FRCOphth

Consultant Ophthalmologist, Aberdeen Royal Hospitals, Aberdeen, UK

CHURCHILL LIVINGSTONE

NEW YORK EDINBURGH LONDON MADRID MELBOURNE SAN FRANCISCO AND TOKYO 1996

CHURCHILL LIVINGSTONE

Medical Division of Pearson Professional Limited

Distributed in the United States of America by Churchill
Livingstone Inc., 650 Avenue of the Americas, New York,
N.Y. 10011, and by associated companies, branches and
representatives throughout the world.

First published 1996

ISBN 0 443 04773 1

British Library Cataloguing in Publication Data
A catalogue record for this book is available from the British
Library.

Library of Congress Cataloging in Publication Data
A catalog record for this book is available from the Library of
Congress.

5/8/96
M

Produced by Longman Singapore Publishers (Pte) Ltd
Printed in Singapore

Contents

Preface

This book is a practical, step-by-step guide to examination techniques in ophthalmic ultrasound. It is primarily aimed at the busy ophthalmologist wanting to perform this investigation as part of the management of his or her own patient. It is also intended as an introductory manual for ophthalmologists, radiologists, radiographers, and other health workers interested in this field, or planning to perform echography on a regular basis.

The emphasis is on how to produce the best pictures (echograms), gather the maximum acoustic data, and interpret the echographic findings. In addition to examination techniques, the book also provides an overview of the clinical application of ultrasound, both in the eye and orbit. Many of these new and exciting applications have only become possible as a result of the recent innovations and developments in instrumentation. Methods of axial eye length measurement (biometry) and corneal thickness (pachymetry) are also described. The book contains references for each chapter, and a glossary of common technical jargon.

Reading this book will not replace 'hands-on' experience. Its purpose will have been achieved, however, if the reader finds it useful in getting started, and thereafter progresses to develop his or her own unique skills.

H. R. Atta

Acknowledgements

The main material included in this book was gathered from my experience in the Echography Clinic, Aberdeen Royal Infirmary. It would not have been possible to set up the ultrasound service and collect this material without the continuing support and encouragement of my consultant colleagues, whom I also thank for allowing me to print clinical material related to their patients.

My initial experience in this field goes back a little further, in particular to a period of training in the Echography Department, Bascom Palmer Eye Institute, Miami, under the supervision of Sandra Frazier Byrne. I am most grateful to her and all the staff in her department for their time and effort in teaching me, and especially to Sandra Byrne for lending me a collection of echographic slides, some of which are presented in the book.

The book contains numerous illustrations, clinical photographs and artist's line drawings. A great deal of time and effort was spent on their production by the staff of the Medical Illustration Department, Medical School, Aberdeen University. In particular I wish to acknowledge the help of Nigel Lukins, Bruce Mireylees, and Alison Farrow.

Finally, thanks to my wife, for her patience and for salvaging the book when a 'digital disaster' nearly wiped it off the computer before we had obtained a hard copy!

H. R. Atta

1

Introduction

INDICATIONS

The application of ultrasonography (echography) in the field of ophthalmic diagnosis has steadily increased over time, being influenced by the availability of superior instruments, improvements in examination techniques, and ever-changing clinical requirements.

Within the last decade, A-scan measurement of axial eye length (biometry) and B-scan screening of the opaque ocular media, particularly in eyes with cataract and vitreous haemorrhage, have constituted the two most common indications for ocular ultrasound examination. A-scan measurement of corneal thickness (pachymetry) is a good example of a new and expanding application of ultrasound, following the introduction of corneal refractive surgery and the consequential need for accurate estimation of corneal thickness. Furthermore, the echographic examination of intraocular lesions, even if they are clearly visible on fundoscopy, has become an essential component in the differentiation of many ocular diseases such as intraocular tumours, leukokorias, macular lesions, optic disc abnormalities, and choroidal folds.

The evaluation of patients undergoing retinal detachment surgery and vitrectomy invariably requires the aid of ultrasonography, as ophthalmoscopy is often hampered by media opacities. Echography in these situations will help the surgeon assess the extent of retinal detachment, the degree and location of vitreo-retinal adhesions, the state of the subretinal space, and the presence and extent of choroidal detachment. In ocular trauma, echography plays an important role in highlighting damage to the posterior segment, and in the detection and localization of intraocular foreign bodies, particularly those that are radiotranslucent.

The echographic investigation of orbital diseases has experienced mixed fortunes. In the late 1960s and early 1970s it was advocated for this purpose. But with the concurrent development of computed tomographic (CT) scanning and, more recently, magnetic resonance imaging (MRI) – both yielding high-quality images of the orbital contents, bony walls, and intracranial compartments – orbital echography has undergone a period of 'recession'. However, within the last few years it has seen a revival, following the development of 'eye-dedicated' B-scanners producing real-time, high-resolution images, and 'standardized' A-scans offering, for the first time, the capability of 'tissue differentiation'. Many subtle orbital abnormalities, such as optic nerve drüsen and sheath distension, enlargement of the extraocular muscles, and engorgement of orbital veins, are better detected on echography. The unique dynamic quality of ultrasound imaging allows the depiction of vascular and pulsatile lesions, and the effect of ocular movements on normal and abnormal orbital structures.

The additional development of Doppler ultrasound, some combined with B-scan (Duplex) and others offering colour coding of blood flow (Colour Doppler), has provided an extra diagnostic tool in the investigation of vascular orbital lesions and abnormalities of ocular circulation.

In the orbit, echography can now be performed either as a primary screening method, to assess the need for further expensive and invasive investigations such as CT and MRI scanning and cerebral angiography, or as a complementary and corroborative test to the above investigations.

HISTORY AND DEVELOPMENT OF OPHTHALMIC ULTRASOUND

The history of 'ultrasound diagnosis' in medicine is relatively short, dating back to the end of the Second World War. The earliest reported application in ophthalmology was by Mundt and Hughes,[1] who in 1956 described the use of pulse-echo (A-scan) technique in the detection of intraocular tumours. Further work on the fundamentals of A-scan diagnosis was carried out by Oksala.[2] The application of A-scan for the purpose of biometry was first described by Gernet in 1965.[3]

Baum and Greenwood developed the first B-scan for ophthalmic use, employing an immersion technique.[4] However, it was not until 1972, when Bronson and Turner produced the first contact B-scan method,[5] that ultrasonography became a more practical investigation. This method made the examination easier to per-

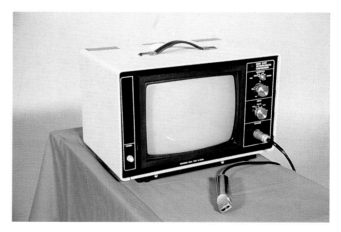

Figure 1.1 Bronson and Turner B-scan. This was the first B-scanner utilizing the 'contact' method. Note the relatively large size of the probe. In spite of this and the low image resolution, the contact method was a major breakthrough in ophthalmic ultrasonography

form, less time-consuming, and more acceptable to patients (Figure 1.1). The popularization and expansion of B-scan technique in the late 1970s is credited to the efforts of Purnell and Coleman.[6,7] In 1964 Buschmann and others founded the International Society for Ophthalmic Ultrasound (SIDUO). This forum, the oldest in any speciality ultrasound, meets biannually and its proceedings are regularly published.

In the meantime, throughout the 1960s and 1970s, painstaking work by Ossoinig and Till in Austria and, later, by Ossoinig in Iowa City, culminated in the development of a highly sophisticated (standardized) A-scan equipment (Figure 1.2), specifically designed for ophthalmic diagnosis.[8,9,10,11] The combination of standardized A-scan, B-scan, and Doppler ultrasound employing well-prescribed examination techniques is collectively known as the method of 'standardized echography'.[12,13]

MODES OF SCANNING

Currently, four diagnostic ultrasound components can be identified in ophthalmology:

1. Biometry A-scan, for axial eye length and corneal pachymetry.
2. Standardized A-scan, for tissue diagnosis.
3. Diagnostic B-scan.
4. Doppler ultrasound.

Throughout this book, all the A-scan examinations, apart from biometry of axial eye length and corneal thickness, were conducted using standardized A-scan instruments, namely the Kretztechnik 7200 MA (Figure 1.2), the Ophthascan-S, and the Ophthascan Mini-A (Figure 1.3). In the text, the term 'A-scan' is synonymous with 'standardized A-scan'.

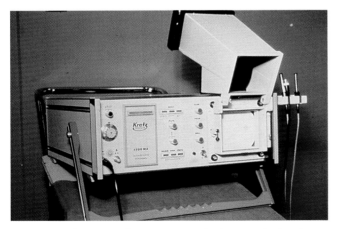

Figure 1.2 The Kretztechnik 7200 MA. The first standardized A-scan, developed by Ossoinig in Austria. Internal and external calibration ensured uniformity of results and reliable comparison and follow-up studies

B-scan examinations were performed using the Ophthascan-S and Ultrascan Digital B System IV (Figures 1.3, 1.4). A hand-held, non-directional Doppler

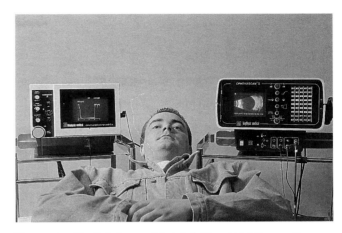

Figure 1.3 The Ophthascan Mini-A (left) and Ophthascan-S (right). Both instruments provide standardized A-scan and facilities for image freeze frame and electronic measuring gates. The Ophthascan-S also provides high-resolution, contact B-scan

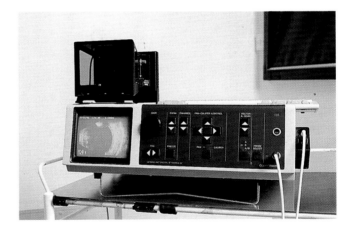

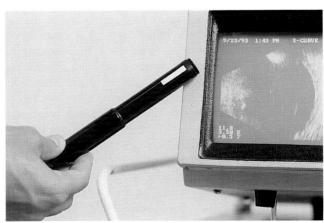

Figure 1.4 The Ultrascan Digital B System IV (top) and its probe (bottom). A fully digitized contact B-scanner, providing computer interface and direct video display capabilities. Note the relatively small size of the probe, allowing flexible manoeuvring and easy access to periphery of the globe

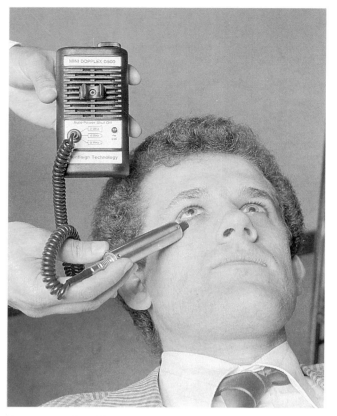

Figure 1.5 A hand-held, non-directional, continuous-wave Doppler instrument for orbital examination

instrument (Figure 1.5) was utilized in orbital examination.

The A- and B-scan pictures (echograms) illustrated are intended to be read from left to right, i.e. the initial spike to the left followed by the anterior segment, vitreous cavity, posterior globe wall, and finally the orbit to the right.

The choice between employing A- or B-scanning mode depends on a number of factors, such as the experience of the examiner, the availability of instruments, and the pertaining clinical situation. Proponents of the two techniques have, in the past, highlighted the virtues of their preferred method and the limitations of the other. It is now recognized, however, that both modalities are essential and complementary if one is to gather the maximum possible acoustic data in order to achieve reliable and accurate results.[12,13,14]

Unlike radiological diagnosis, echography requires the examiner to be skilled in both the acquisition of images and interpretation of the results, since the diagnosis is mainly obtained during the dynamic scanning and not from still pictures. Therefore, the role of 'radiographer' and 'radiologist' has to merge into one in the echographic investigation. As a result, a need exists for ophthalmologists, who want to perform this technique, to train in the basic principles of ultrasound

physics and examination methods, and for 'non-ophthalmic echographers' to acquire sufficient knowledge in the basic science and disease process in ophthalmology. In addition, the satisfactory training of personnel necessitates the introduction of a structured protocol for examination. This is also a prerequisite for the conducting of accurate follow-up and research studies.

Recent advances in instrument design and development have resulted in a vast improvement in the quality of images, mostly captured in real-time scanning. Other welcome facilities include colour coding, three-dimensional creation, image freeze frame, electronic measuring gates, video display, and digital storage. Arguably more suitable than other imaging modalities, echography is now utilized for tissue differentiation of lesions. Some of the most recent and exciting innovations include the introduction of ultrasound contrast media and the development of high-frequency, microscopic, B-scan images of the anterior segment structures, the so-called 'ultrasound biomicroscopy'.[15]

Finally, the non-invasive and cost-effective nature of ultrasound gives it an additional and distinct advantage over other imaging modalities. This will ensure its prominent role in ophthalmic and other fields of medical diagnosis for many years to come.

REFERENCES

1 Mundt G H, Hughes W E. Ultrasonics in ocular diagnosis. Am J Ophthalmol 1956; 41:488–498

2 Oksala A, Lehtinen A. Diagnostic value of ultrasonics in ophthalmology. Ophthalmologica 1957; 134:387–395 (In German)

3 Gernet H. Biometrie des Auges mit Ultraschall. Klin Monatsbl Augenheilkd 1965; 146:863–874

4 Baum G, Greenwood I. The application of ultrasonic locating techniques to ophthalmology: theoretic considerations and acoustic properties of ocular media: Part 1. Reflective properties. Am J Ophthalmol 1958; 46:319–329

5 Bronson N R, Turner F T. A simple B-scan ultrasonoscope. Arch Ophthalmol 1973; 90:237–238

6 Purnell E W. B-mode orbital ultrasonography. Int Ophthalmol Clin 1969; 9:643–665

7 Coleman D J, Lizzi F L, Jack R L. Ultrasonography of the eye and orbit. Philadelphia: Lea & Febiger, 1977

8 Ossoinig K C. Standardized echography: basic principles, clinical applications and results. Int Ophthalmol Clin. 1979; 19:127–210

9 Till P, Ossoinig K C. 10 years' study on clinical echography in intraocular diseases. Bibl Ophthalmol 1975; 83:49–62

10 Ossoinig K C. Quantitative echography – the basis of tissue differentiation. J Clin Ultrasound 1974; 2:33–46

11 Ossoinig K C. New apparatus for echographic diagnosis in ophthalmology. Graefes Arch Ophthalmol 1967; 171:312–317 (In German)

12 Byrne S F, Green R L. Ultrasound of the eye and orbit. St Louis: Mosby Year Book, 1992

13 Byrne S F. Standardized echography of the eye and orbit. Neuroradiology 1986; 28:618–640

14 Atta H R. Techniques and application of diagnostic ultrasound. In: Easty D L (ed) Current ophthalmic surgery. London: Baillière Tindall, 1990:31–46

15 Pavlin C J, Sherar M D, Harasiewicz K. et al Clinical use of ultrasound biomicroscopy. Ophthalmology 1991; 98:287–295

2

Echographic examination: general principles

In this chapter a brief description is given of the general requirements for ultrasound examination. These are based on the author's own experience, and accordingly represent only guidelines. Other examiners may choose different practices that reflect their own hospital environment, speciality interest, the volume of service, and the availability of instruments.

ORGANIZATION OF ULTRASOUND CLINIC

In large departments, where one examiner is likely to be responsible for providing the ultrasound service, it is advisable to dedicate a number of fixed 'clinic sessions' to such a purpose. This is to facilitate the structured training of personnel and permit adequate time for documentation, reporting, and filing. An ultrasound request form is best introduced in order to improve referral patterns (Figure 2.1). This should include patient data, summary of clinical presentation, and, most importantly, the specific question(s) to be answered by the ultrasound examination. A report giving the findings and 'clinical impression' should be furnished on completion of the examination.

Although knowledge of the clinical features is always helpful, the examiner ought not to be biased by it. The 'echographic' diagnosis should be reached primarily from the acoustic data collected during the dynamic scanning.

EXAMINATION ROOM

Echography should be conducted in a separate, quiet room, with facilities for dim lighting. The room must be well ventilated, as equipment tends to generate heat. A reclining, swivel chair with height and tilt adjustment is best provided for the patient; this is better than the ubiquitous couch with its uncomfortable flat lie. In addition, an overhead, mobile fixation light is helpful in directing the patient's gaze to the required position. This, as will be discussed later, is essential for placing lesions in the centre (most sensitive part) of the echogram, and for accurate biometric measurement of structures such as tumour height and diameter of the optic nerve and extraocular muscles. Ultrasound equipment needs to be placed on a suitable movable working surface, for flexibility and ease of access.

The following are also required for echographic examination: coupling ultrasound jelly, topical anaesthetic, alcohol wipes, sterile saline for irrigation, and, finally, an ample supply of paper tissues, all placed within easy reach of the examiner. The tip of some B-scan probes requires periodic filling with water to eliminate air bubbles. Only distilled water – not saline – should be used, otherwise damage to the cap and rubber components will result from salt erosion.

Depending on the instrument used, various recording facilities are needed, e.g. Polaroid and 35 mm cameras with appropriate films, video recorder, display, and printer. Modern scanners may also allow computer storage and retrieval of images.

EXAMINATION STEPS

The procedure is first explained to the patient, with emphasis on the safety and harmless nature of ultrasound. The patient is then seated on the reclining chair, with the examiner (if right-handed) positioned to the right of the patient. The instrument display

ECHOGRAPHY REQUEST FORM

Patient's name _____ Unit No. _____

Age _____ Consultant _____ Date _____

Any previous echography   Yes ☐   No ☐

Diagnosis

Evaluate   RE   LE

Visual acuity   RE_____ LE_____ IOP   RE____ LE ____

Exophthalmometry   RE ___   LE ___   Base _____

Relevant history and Clinical findings _____

_____

_____

_____

Are there specific questions you wanted answered? _____

_____

Location of Fundus Lesion

Equator

Referred by _____

Figure 2.1 An example of an ultrasound request form. The referring physician is invited to be specific about the reason for the request and the information required from the ultrasound examination

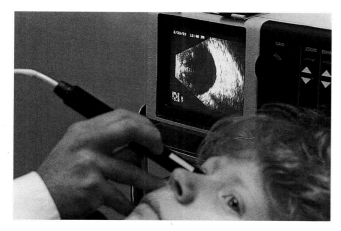

Figure 2.2 Ultrasound examination is best carried out with the patient in the reclining position and the head as near as possible to the instrument's screen. The examiner is thus able to observe the probe position on the eye and the echogram image with ease

Table 2.1 Methodology and instrumentation in ocular echography	
Data	Scanning mode
I Screening	**B-scan**
Lesion detected?-----> No	End of examination
Lesion detected?-----> Yes	Proceed............
II Topographic examination	
Shape	B-scan
Location	B-scan
Extension	B-scan
III Quantitative examination	
Reflectivity	A- and B-scans
Texture	A-scan
Sound attenuation	A-scan
IV Kinetic examination	
Mobility	B-scan
After-movement	A- and B-scans
Vascularity	A-scan
'Echographic diagnosis'	

screen is brought as near to the patient's head as possible. The examiner is then able to observe the screen and probe orientation with ease (Figure 2.2).

Both A- and B-mode scanning are invariably required to collect the maximum acoustic information.

In some instances, B-scan alone is sufficient, e.g. in screening an eye with dense cataract where no other abnormalities are detected. Equally, A-scan is adequate for screening the orbit and for measuring the width of the optic nerve and extraocular muscles. In general, B-scan is more applicable in ocular examination, particularly vitreo-retinal disorders, while A-scan is more sensitive in detecting orbital diseases, especially those involving the optic nerve and extra ocular muscles. Doppler ultrasound is occasionally used to assess the vascularity of lesions and detect increased blood flow in the orbit. More sophisticated Doppler instruments incorporating colour coding and simultaneous B-scan display are now increasingly used for ophthalmic evaluation.

A systematic approach to echographic examination is recommended if reliable and reproducible results are to be obtained. This is outlined by the following steps:

1. Screening, for lesion detection.
2. Topographic examination, i.e. shape, border, and location of lesion.
3. Quantitative echography, i.e. reflectivity, sound attenuation, and internal structure of lesion.
4. Kinetic echography, i.e. mobility, vascularity, and consistency of lesion.

As an example, let us say that during *screening* of the globe a membranous opacity is detected in the vitreous cavity. The membrane takes the configuration of an open funnel, occupying four quadrants, and is attached to the optic nerve (*topographic data*). The membrane has a limited mobility (*kinetic data*) and exhibits a bright appearance on B-scan and a high A-scan spike equal to that of sclera (*quantitative data*). The above findings are consistent with the diagnosis of retinal detachment.

The echographer, depending on the nature of the examination, will perform the above steps in various orders and degrees of detail before reaching the correct diagnosis and supplying the referring physician with the maximum possible information. Lastly, the findings are documented.

Table 2.1 summarizes the four components of ultrasound examination and the recommended scanning mode for collecting the relevant acoustic data.

THE GLOBE

3

Ocular screening

OCULAR SCREENING: A-SCAN

General principles

An understanding of the factors which determine the appearance of tissue signals during A-scan examination is essential in order to provide the examiner with the required knowledge to perform the examination and interpret the results correctly.

A-scan (A for amplitude) provides a one-dimensional display of returning echoes in the form of vertical spikes of various heights and distances from the initial signal. The A-scan appearance of a normal eye is illustrated in Figure 3.1.

Two fundamental data are obtained from A-scan examination:

1. The distance of echo-source from the probe face. This forms the basis of 'biometry'.
2. The amplitude of echo-signal (spike), which partly depends on the nature of the reflecting interface. This forms the basis of 'quantitative echography'.

It is important to recognize that the distance and height of a spike depend not only on the location and nature of the echo-source, i.e. 'tissue factors', but also on the energy (decibel) gain and the direction of the sound beam, i.e. 'external factors'.

A beam aimed perpendicularly on a reflecting surface produces the strongest signal in the shortest distance (Figure 3.2), whilst a direct relation exists

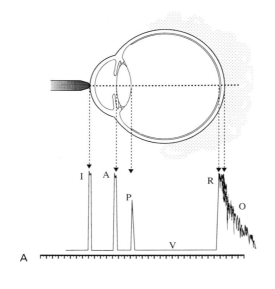

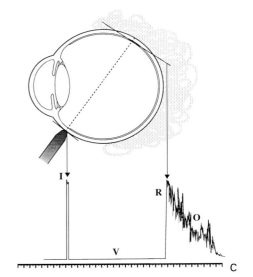

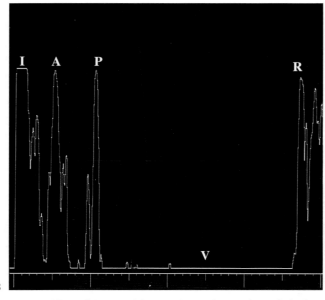

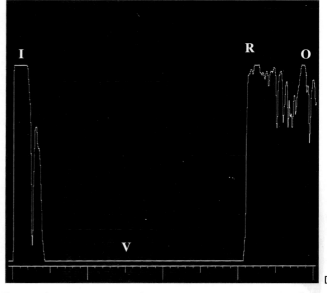

Figure 3.1 Normal A-scan of the eye. An axial scan (through the lens) is illustrated in Figures 3.1A and 3.1B. A posterior scan (avoiding the lens), often required to improve resolution and maintain perpendicular beam incidence, is shown in Figures 3.1C and 3.1D. I = initial spike, A = anterior lens/iris spike, P = posterior lens spike, V = vitreous 'base line', R = retinal spike, O = orbital spikes

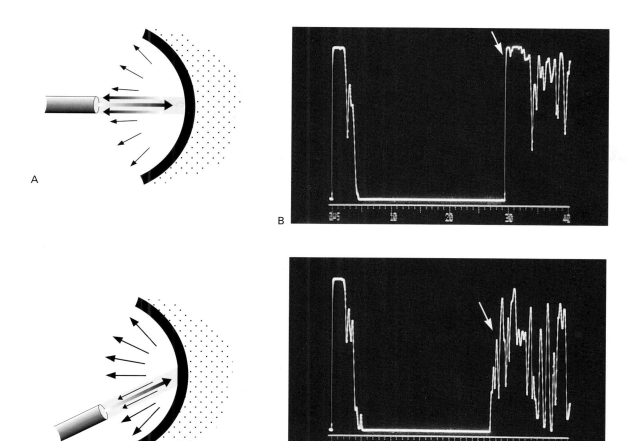

Figure 3.2 Effect of perpendicularity on the appearance of A-scan signals. A beam aligned perpendicularly on the globe wall allows the maximum amount of echoes (energy) to return to the transducer (Figure 3.2A), resulting in the strongest retinal signal (arrow) (Figure 3.2B). An oblique beam incidence results in greater loss of returning echoes from refraction and reflection (Figure 3.2C) and a weaker, jagged retinal spike (arrow) (Figure 3.2D)

between the decibel gain and spike height (Figure 3.3). Other factors influencing spike characteristics include sound impedance and beam scatter, which in turn depend on the nature of the tissues. Sound reflection and refraction are determined by the angle of the incident beam.

The reliable 'tissue diagnosis' of lesions on A-scan depends, therefore, on the standardization of equipment and examination methods, that minimalizes the influence of 'external factors'.

Standardization of A-scan

It is now recognized by workers in this field that standardization of instruments and examination methods is essential for diagnostic A-scanning, as it permits the reliable interpretation of echo-signals and accurate comparison and quantification of results.

The development of a standardized A-scan for ophthalmic diagnosis is credited to the work of Dr Karl Ossoinig.[1,2,3,4,5] The first commercially available instrument, the Kretztechnik (Figure 1.2), was manufactured in Austria in the late 1960s. In the last few

years, this equipment has been superseded by the Ophthascan-S, the Ophthascan Mini-A (Figure 1.3), and other 'standardized' A-scan equipment, most combined with B-scan and biometry facilities – e.g. Bio-vision (BV International, France).

In addition to a uniform internal design, all standardized A-scans contain the following features:

1. Unique sound amplification (Figure 3.4): an S-shaped amplifier with flat upper and lower curves and a steep mid segment, and a dynamic range of 36 dB. This amplification enhances the difference between normal and abnormal signals.[5,6]

2. Probe design (Figure 3.3): an 8 MHz pencil-size probe, emitting parallel sound beam. The beam width varies from 5.0 mm at its highest decibel gain to 0.5 mm at its lowest. The non-focused A-scan beam is considered important in determining perpendicularity.

3. Tissue model: a 'phantom', supplied by the manufacturer, which enables the examiner to calibrate the instrument to the desired tissue sensitivity gain (T-sensitivity). This is a moderately

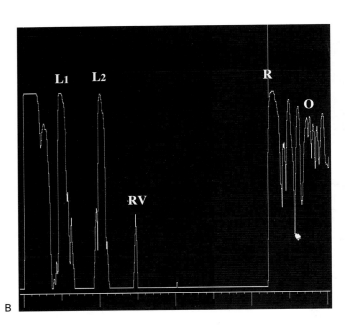

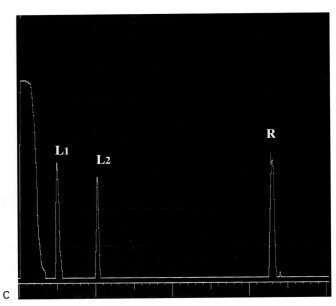

Figure 3.3 Effect of decibel (dB) gain on the appearance of A-scan signals. Figure 3.3A illustrates the profile of the A-scan beam at a high decibel gain (wide grey line) and a low gain (narrow black line). In Figure 3.3B, the A-scan trace is taken at a high dB level. Compare the height and thickness of lens (L1 and L2) and retinal (R) spikes to that in Figure 3.3C, taken at a low dB gain. The reverberation signal (RV) and orbital spikes (O) have disappeared in the low gain trace

high decibel gain providing optimum tissue differentiation.[7,8] Identifying T-sensitivity for each probe/instrument combination is an essential component of standardization, as it ensures the uniform appearance of the same lesion with various instruments. The examiner may, as will be seen later, employ higher or lower gain settings during examination, as dictated by the individual case. Once established, T-sensitivity needs to be

Figure 3.4 Sound amplification curves. Linear amplification provides high sensitivity and low dynamic range (useful in biometry); the opposite applies to the logarithmic curve. S-shaped amplification is an optimal compromise allowing adequate sensitivity and a wide range of amplitude amplification. (Reproduced with permission from Ossoinig K C Standardized Echography: basic principles, clinical applications, and results. Int Ophthalmol Clinics 19:127–210 1979)

verified only occasionally or if the probe is renewed. The setting of T-sensitivity is summarized in Figure 3.5.

Examination steps

A methodical approach to examination techniques is fundamental to standardization process. The recommended steps are as follows:

1. The instrument is set at T-sensitivity (Figure 3.5).
2. The patient is positioned with the head near the oscilloscope.
3. Topical anaesthetic drops are placed in the eye.
4. The probe is placed firmly on the globe (Figure 3.6). No coupling jelly is required, as the tear film acts as an adequate sound-transmitting medium.
5. Eight meridians are scanned, postero-anteriorly (Figure 3.7), by shifting and tilting the probe in a single, smooth arc movement from limbus to fornix. To help maintain perpendicular beam incidence on the ocular wall, the patient is instructed to gaze towards the meridian to be scanned, aided by the fixation light. In all scans, perpendicularity of the beam incidence is verified by the observation of a smooth, steeply rising, tall retinal spike (Figure 3.2).

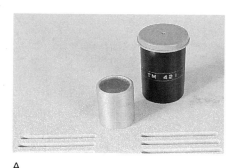

A

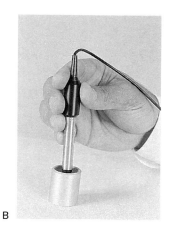

B

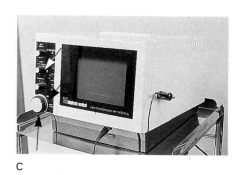

C

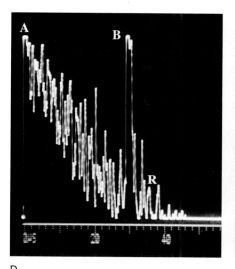

D

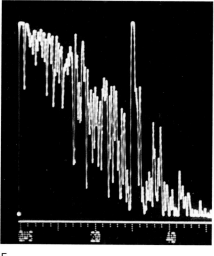

E

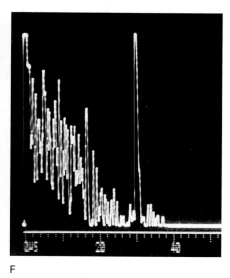

F

Figure 3.5 The setting of 'tissue (T) sensitivity'. Figure 3.5A: a tissue model (TM) is supplied by the manufacturer for the purpose of calibration of T-sensitivity. Figure 3.5B: the A-scan probe is placed vertically on the surface of TM after application of a coupling jelly. Figure 3.5C: the display is switched to 'orbit' using the appropriate button (top arrow), and the dB level is altered using the dB control switch (bottom arrow). Figure 3.5D, 3.5E, and 3.5F illustrate the appearance of trace at three different dB levels. As the sound travels through the TM, the echoes decline from left to right, forming an N-shaped pattern with the TM surface spike (A) and bottom spike (B); R = reverberation signals. The T-sensitivity level is obtained when an equal N-shaped pattern is produced, as in Figure 3.5D. T + 6 gain and T − 6 gain are illustrated in Figures 3.5E and 3.5F respectively

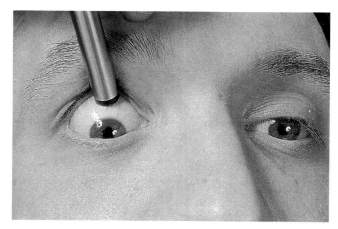

Figure 3.6 A-scanning is conducted through open lids. Firm contact between probe tip and the globe ensures good sound transmission.

6. Depending on the requirements of each examination, the scanning of four or eight meridians is repeated using a higher level of decibels – e.g. T plus 6 – to detect fine vitreous opacities (Figure 3.8) and a lower level – e.g. T minus 24 – to measure retino-choroid layer thickness and height of mass lesions, and to isolate high foreign body signal (Figure 3.9).

7. In some circumstances, such as with traumatized or infected eyes, or soon after intraocular surgery, examination through closed eyelids is safer. To maintain standardization in these cases, 3 decibels are added to T-sensitivity to compensate for energy absorbed by scanning through the skin.

8. At the end of the procedure, the eye is irrigated with sterile saline, and the probe tip is cleansed

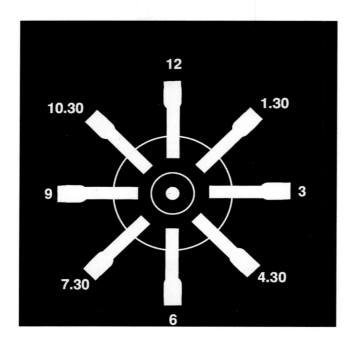

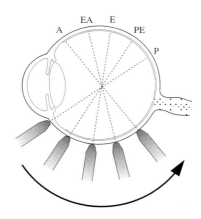

Figure 3.7 Eight 'clock-hours' meridians are scanned postero-anteriorly, by shifting and rotating the probe (antero-posteriorly) from limbus to fornix (A = anterior, E = equator, P = posterior.)

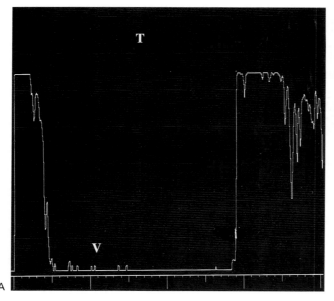

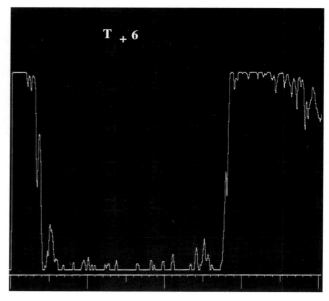

Figure 3.8 High (T + 6) gain is employed to demonstrate fine vitreous opacities. Figure 3.8A is a trace taken at T sensitivity, showing few insignificant spikes (mostly noise echoes) in the vitreous (V). In Figure 3.8B, taken at T + 6 sensitivity, a series of short spikes occupies the entire vitreous base line, indicating fine dispersed vitreous opacities, such as fresh blood or inflammatory cells

with alcohol wipe or another suitable disinfectant. The probe can be sterilized – e.g. following examination of endophthalmitis cases – by immersing it in a disinfectant solution for the recommended duration.

Orientation and labelling of scans

Once a lesion has been detected, precise localization of its position is undertaken by observing the meridian and antero-posterior location of the probe on the globe wall. The labelling of sections is determined by the projection of the beam and not the probe location. For example, a section labelled 12 equator (12E) (Figure 3.10) is produced by placing the probe at 6 o'clock, mid-distance between limbus and fornix. A section labelled 6 anterior (6A) (Figure 3.11) is produced by placing the probe at 12 o'clock fornix, and section 3 posterior (3P) (Figure 3.12) is the result of a probe positioned at 9 o'clock limbus.

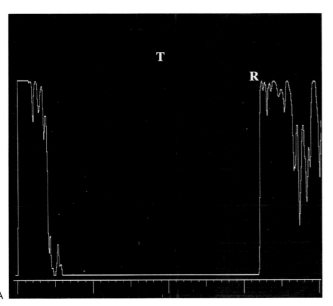

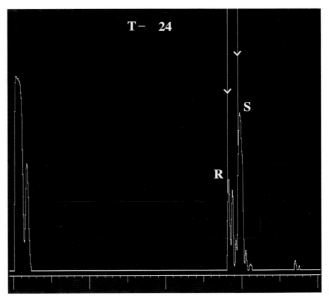

A

B

Figure 3.9 Low (T − 24) gain used to examine and measure the chorio-retinal layer. Figure 3.9A is a T-sensitivity trace in a normal eye. The retinal spike (R) is indistinguishable from that of the sclera. In Figure 3.9B, the gain is lowered while maintaining perpendicularity. The retinal spike is clearly visible (R) and is separated from the scleral spike (S) by a distance of 1.05 mm. The short spike between R and S represents the choroid. The two vertical lines (arrows) indicate the position of the electronic measuring gates

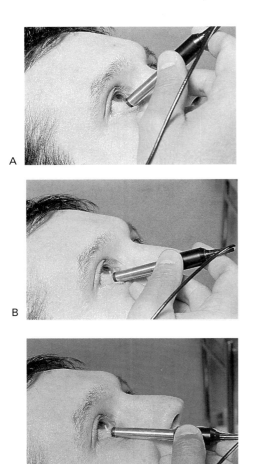

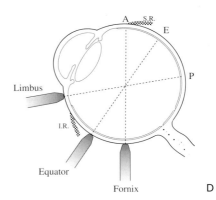

Figure 3.10 A-scanning of 12 o'clock fundus. Probe is placed at 6 o'clock limbus for 12P (Figure 3.10A), at equator for 12E (Figure 3.10B), and at fornix for 12A (Figure 3.10C). The probe and beam orientation are schematically drawn in Figure 3.10D. S.R. = superior rectus muscle; I.R. = inferior rectus muscle.

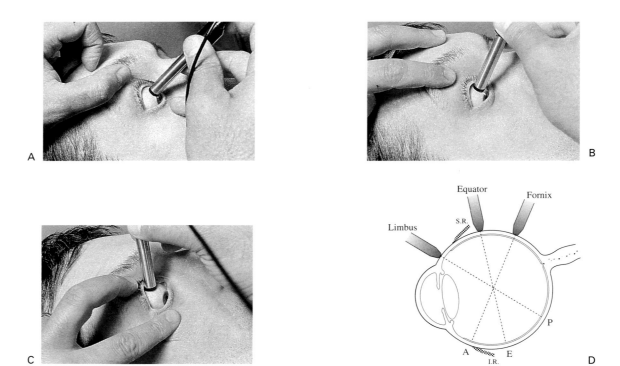

Figure 3.11 A-scanning of 6 o'clock fundus. Probe is placed at 12 o'clock limbus, equator and fornix for posterior, equator and anterior sections respectively (Figures 3.11A, 3.11B, and 3.11C). These are further illustrated in Figure 3.11D

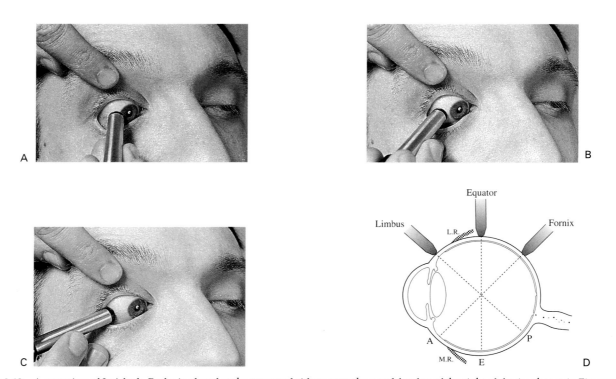

Figure 3.12 A-scanning of 3 o'clock. Probe is placed at the temporal side to scan the nasal fundus of the right globe (as shown in Figures 3.12A, 3.12B, 3.12C, and 3.12D). For the left eye, the probe would be placed nasally to scan the temporal fundus. L.R. = lateral rectus muscle; M.R. = medial rectus muscle.

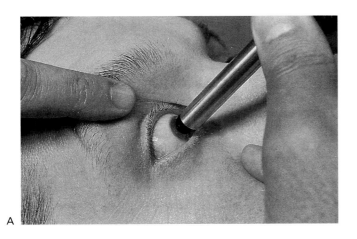

A

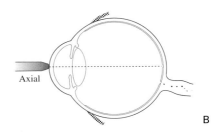

Axial

B

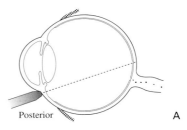

C

Figure 3.13 Axial screening of the macula. In Figure 3.13A, the probe is placed on the anaesthetized cornea. Figure 3.13B illustrates the beam path. Figure 3.13C shows the appearance of the A-scan trace. L = anterior and posterior lens spikes, RV = reverberation artefact, M = macular signal

Macular screening

Lesions at the macula need to be measured and differentiated. Two approaches are available for such purposes: axial and posterior.

1. Axial section (Figure 3.13). This is the easier of the two approaches. The probe is placed on the cornea and directed axially. A small amount of coupling jelly may be applied on the probe tip to prevent corneal abrasion. Perpendicular and axial beam orientation is confirmed when tall anterior and posterior lens and retinal spikes are produced. Although suitable for measurements, this section is not sensitive in detecting early macular thickening or in the differentiation of its lesions, because of the strong sound attenuation by the lens.
2. Posterior section (Figure 3.14). In the right eye this is the 9P position and in the left the 3P position. It is produced by directing the patient's gaze temporally and placing the probe at the nasal limbus and aiming it posteriorly, thus avoiding the lens and achieving better resolution and more reliable tissue differentiation.

Examination of fundus periphery

The small, pencil-size, A-scan probe is easy to manoeuvre, allowing the examiner to sweep the sound beam into the periphery of the fundus and ciliary body. The patient's gaze is directed maximally towards the meridian to be scanned, and the probe is placed at the opposite fornix, the beam being aimed across the globe towards the opposite periphery. Perpendicular incidence of the beam may be difficult to maintain, how-

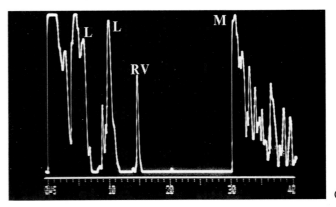

Posterior

A

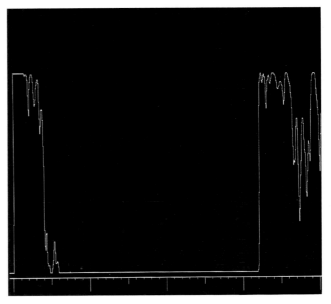

B

Figure 3.14 Macular screening, posterior approach. Figure 3.14A illustrates the beam orientation. By avoiding the lens it is possible to improve resolution. The echogram is shown in Figure 3.14B

19

ever, and, once it reaches the ciliary body, the smooth 'retinal' spike becomes jagged owing to the irregularity of the ciliary body's surface (Figure 3.15).

This scan is useful for detecting peripheral retinal cysts/retino-schisis, choroidal detachments, and ciliary body lesions.

Occasionally, lesions at the extreme inferior and temporal periphery are difficult to scan, as the superior orbital rim and nose, respectively, may prevent full angulation of the probe. Such lesions can be alternatively scanned by placing the probe on the sclera, directly over the lesion at the corresponding meridian. In these cases lesion spikes are displayed immediately after the initial signal (Figure 3.16).

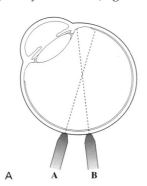

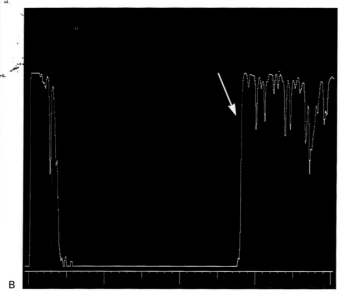

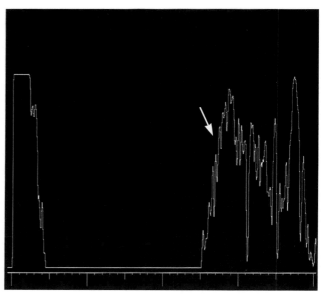

Figure 3.15 A-scanning of fundus periphery. Figure 3.15A is an illustration of the beam orientation. In position A the beam is scanning 'smooth' retinal periphery, producing a tall smooth retinal spike (arrow, Figure 3.15B). In position B, the beam is shifted more peripherally. The 'irregular' ciliary body appears as a jagged spike (arrow, Figure 3.15C)

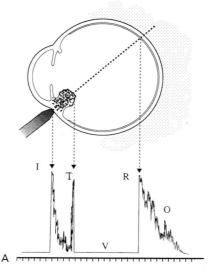

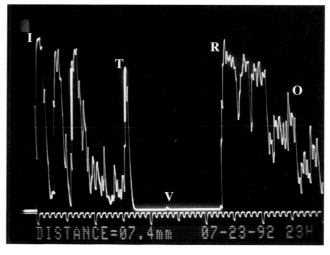

Figure 3.16 Direct A-scanning of retinal periphery and ciliary body. Figure 3.16A shows the beam orientation and the resulting A-scan trace of a ciliary body lesion. Figure 3.16B is an A-scan echogram of a ciliary body melanoma. I = initial spike, T = posterior tumour surface spike, V = vitreous, R = retina at the opposite globe wall, O = orbital spikes)

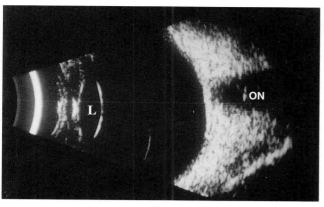

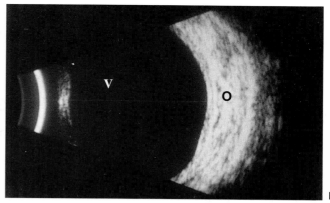

Figure 3.17 Normal contact B-scan of the eye. In Figure 3.17A, the beam travels axially through the lens (L) and optic nerve (ON). In Figure 3.17B, the lens and optic nerve are avoided. V = vitreous cavity, O = orbital cavity

OCULAR SCREENING: B-SCAN

General principles

Unlike the one-dimensional images produced by the non-focused A-scan beam, the B-scan (B for brightness) produces two-dimensional slice-of-tissue images, composed of coalescing dots of varying degrees of brightness, depending on the reflectivity of the echo-source (Figure 3.17). The probe emits a focused sound beam, akin to slit lamp light at a frequency of 10 MHz (Figure 3.18). The 'eye-dedicated' scanners produce a sound beam whose focal zone coincides with the posterior globe wall and anterior orbit. In most scanners, the lateral sweep of the beam is such that it can only scan adequately from equator to equator. Scanning of the periphery, therefore, necessitates shifting the probe and/or patient's gaze to bring lesions into the central, most sensitive part of the beam path and echogram (Figure 3.19).

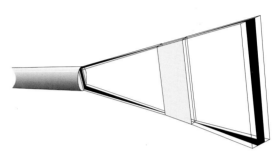

Figure 3.18 Profile of the B-scan beam. In eye-dedicated scanners a focal zone (shaded segment) coincides with the posterior globe wall and anterior orbit for maximum resolution. The (dB) gain affects the width of the beam, which is thick (white outline) at high gain and thin (black outline) at low gain

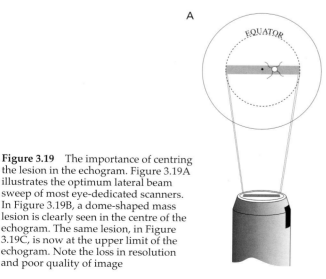

Figure 3.19 The importance of centring the lesion in the echogram. Figure 3.19A illustrates the optimum lateral beam sweep of most eye-dedicated scanners. In Figure 3.19B, a dome-shaped mass lesion is clearly seen in the centre of the echogram. The same lesion, in Figure 3.19C, is now at the upper limit of the echogram. Note the loss in resolution and poor quality of image

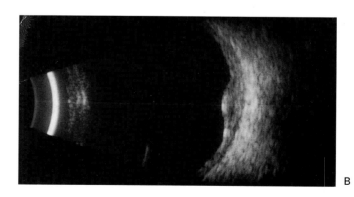

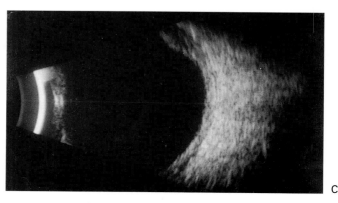

21

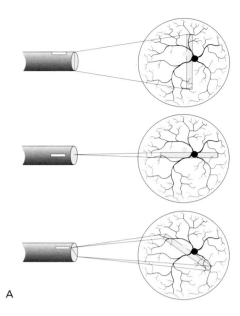

A

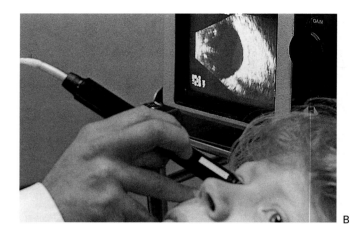

B

Figure 3.20 A marker at the probe tip gives the orientation of the B-scan beam (Figure 3.20A). It also indicates the top of the echogram on the display screen (Figure 3.20B)

A marker at the probe tip indicates the beam orientation and the top of the echogram as it displays on the screen (Figure 3.20). Most of the eye-dedicated instruments also display the echograms with the anterior eye segment to the left and posterior segment and orbit to the right.

As with A-scanning, B-scanning is best conducted directly on the globe to improve resolution and determine the patient's gaze. Care must be taken with traumatized eyes, however, since examining through open eyelids may cause further trauma or introduce an infection. A coupling jelly is applied to the probe tip to ensure adequate sound transmission (Figure 3.21). The probe is cleansed with an alcohol wipe at the end of each examination. For the examination of endophthalmitis cases, coupling jelly can be first applied to the probe tip, and the probe is then covered in 'cling film' or a similar membrane. Impregnating B-probes in sterilizing solution is not recommended, as it may damage the transducer.

Three fundamental objectives need to be fulfilled if high-quality B-scans are to be obtained:

1. Lesions must be placed in the centre of the scanning beam.
2. The beam must be directed perpendicularly to interfaces at the area of interest.
3. The lowest possible decibel gain that is consistent with the maintenance of adequate intensity should be used to optimize resolution of images.

Instrument's control panel

Whereas in A-scan calibration of the decibel gain is the main function on the control panel, B-scan images can be altered in a number of ways to enhance the image quality. These include decibel gain, grey scale, and anterior shift.

1. Decibel gain

No T-sensitivity is needed in B-scanning, as the operator is free to set the level best suited to the individual examination. In general, the lower the gain required to show a lesion, the better the resolution. High gain is normally employed during the initial screening to show fine vitreous opacities and posterior vitreous detachment. Low gain is used to delineate the retinochoroid layer, outline configuration of ocular tumours and detect their extrascleral extension, highlight optic

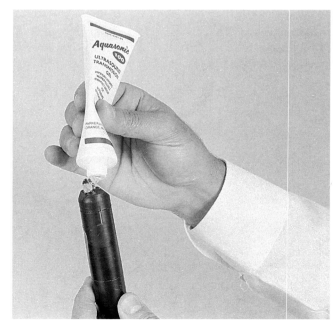

Figure 3.21 An ultrasound coupling jelly being applied on the probe tip. A thick, non-drip solution is preferred

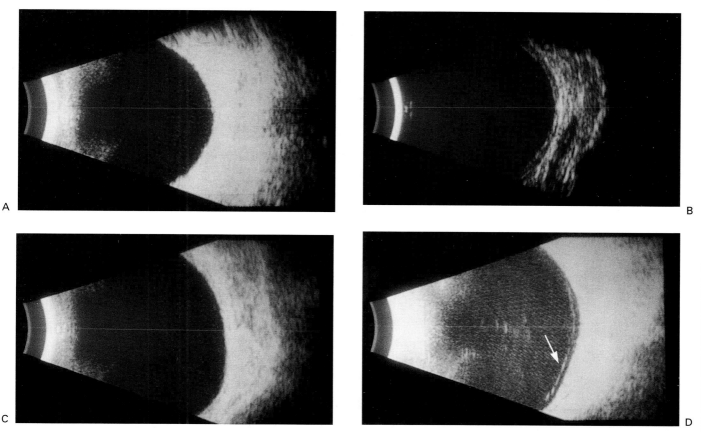

Figure 3.22 Effect of decibel gain on the appearance of a B-scan echogram. Figure 3.22A is a high-gain echogram. In Figure 3.22B, the same segment is scanned using very low gain: the chorio-retinal layer is now highlighted. Figure 3.22C is another medium/high-gain scan; the vitreous cavity appears normal. In Figure 3.22D, the same eye is scanned with maximum gain. A fine, shallow posterior vitreous detachment is detected (arrow)

disc drüsen, and demonstrate calcification in retinoblastoma and intraocular foreign bodies. A high setting followed by a low setting routine is recommended for ocular screening (Figure 3.22).

2. Grey scale

From black to white, the reflectivity of echo-sources is displayed in dots of numerous shades of grey. The higher the instrument's grey scale, the more numerous the shades of grey displayed. In general, it is best to begin scanning with the highest scale to enhance the diagnostic capability of the instrument. For the purposes of documentation and picture quality, it is often necessary to reduce the grey scale, thus creating more contrast (Figure 3.23).

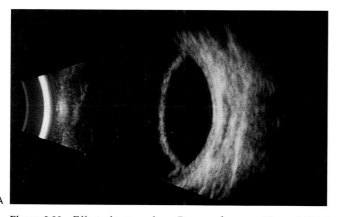 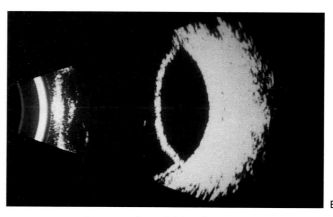

Figure 3.23 Effect of grey scale on B-scan echogram. Figure 3.23A is a low-contrast scan of a serous choroidal detachment. In Figure 3.23B, the scale is reduced, creating more contrast and improving the pictorial appeal of the image

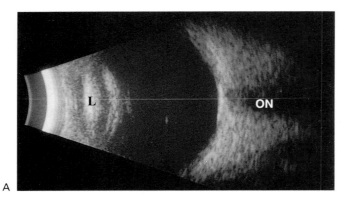

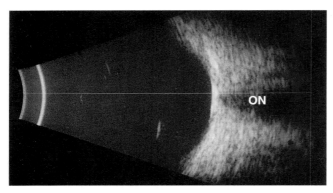

Figure 3.24 Effect of 'anterior shift'. In Figure 3.24A, the anterior (left) portion of the echogram is maximally displayed. In Figure 3.24B it is maximally inhibited. No significant loss of resolution is noted in the posterior segment. L = lens, ON = optic nerve

3. Anterior shift

This function selectively suppresses the anterior segment of the echogram, on the assumption that inhibiting this portion improves the resolution of the posterior segment, where most of the lesions are likely to be located. The author did not find this to be significant in the instruments used. Displaying the anterior segment is, however, important in some circumstances, e.g. for detecting lens lesions (rupture or foreign body), cyclitic membrane, and anterior vitreous opacities (Figure 3.24).

B-scan sections: orientation and labelling

Three basic sections are obtained from B-scanning: axial, transverse, and longitudinal.

1. Axial section

This is the easiest to perform and interpret. The patient fixates at the primary gaze and the probe is placed on the cornea and directed axially. In this section the posterior lens surface and optic nerve head are placed in

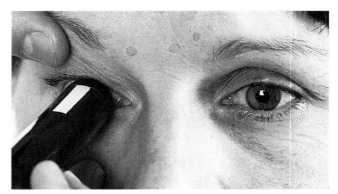

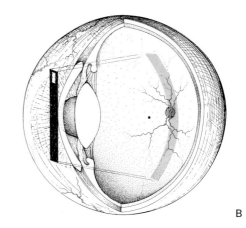

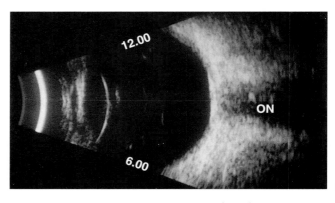

Figure 3.25 Vertical axial B-scan section of the right eye. In Figure 3.25A, the patient directs the gaze at the primary position and the probe is placed on the cornea with its marker at 12 o'clock. Figure 3.25B shows beam orientation. Figure 3.25C gives the actual display, showing the lens (L) and optic nerve (ON) in the centre of the echogram

the centre of the echogram. Although not truly an 'anatomical centre', the optic nerve head, being a good landmark, is conveniently used as the 'echographic centre'. Depending on the clock-hour location of the probe marker, a vertical axial section (marker at 12 o'clock) (Figure 3.25), horizontal axial section (marker at 3 o'clock right eye and 9 o'clock left eye)

(Figure 3.26), and sections of all other clock hours can be performed (Figure 3.27).

Axial sections are used for easy orientation and demonstration of posterior pole lesions and attachment of membranes to the optic nerve head. But, because of the scatter and strong sound attenuation created by the lens, higher decibel gain levels are needed to show structures at the posterior segment. This is done at the expense of image resolution. Unless they are extremely large, peripheral lesions are also likely to be missed or partially displayed on this sec-

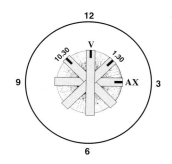
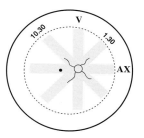

Figure 3.27 Axial B-scanning: the diagram illustrates probe location and beam orientation in axial sections. Any clock-hour meridian can be scanned. In practice, however, only the 'upper' clock hours need to be scanned, as scanning the lower ones would produce the same echogram upside down

tion. In pseudophakic eyes, strong artefacts, created by the lens implant, will hamper adequate visualization.

2. Transverse section

In this section the beam traverses many meridians. But, unlike in the axial section, scanning through the lens is avoided (Figure 3.28). The probe is placed on the limbus and directed posteriorly. In a single smooth arc movement, it is shifted and rotated from limbus to fornix, scanning the opposite globe wall postero-

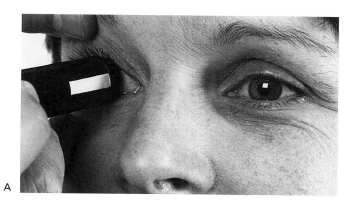

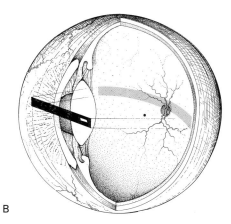

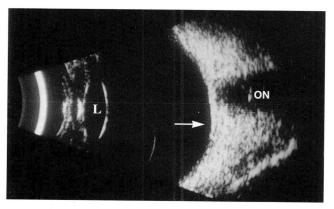

Figure 3.26 Horizontal axial B-scan of the right eye. In Figure 3.26A, the probe is directed axially with its marker at 3 o'clock (nasally). Figure 3.26B is a diagrammatic illustration of beam orientation. Figure 3.26C shows the actual display; the arrow points at the macula

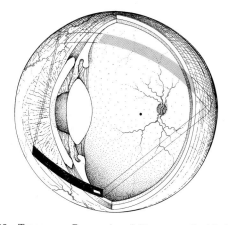

Figure 3.28 Transverse B-scanning, 3-D concept. In this diagram a '12 o'clock-equator' section is produced. The probe is centred half-way between inferior limbus and fornix with its marker nasally, thus projecting a beam at the superior fundal equator, which is centred at 12 o'clock

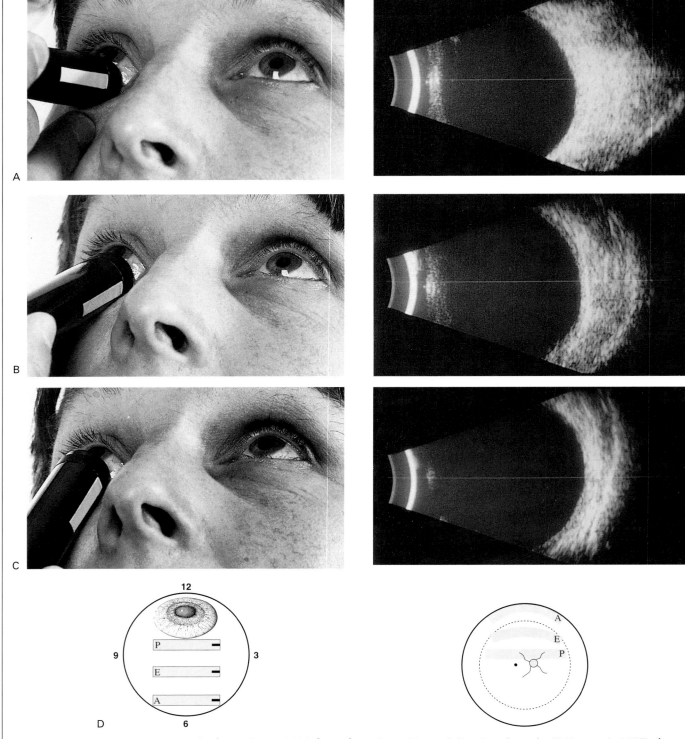

Figure 3.29 Transverse-12 B-scan of right eye. Figure 3.29A shows the probe position and direction of gaze for 'T-12 posterior' (12P); the resulting echogram appears on the right. Figure 3.29 B gives those for 'T-12 equator' (12E), and Figure 3.29C those for 'T-12 anterior' (12A). Note the marker location and probe angle on the eye. Also compare the antero-posterior width of the orbital fact segment in the echograms, which decreases as the eye is scanned more anteriorly. The probe and marker location on the eye, and corresponding beam orientation on the fundus, are also illustrated in Figure 3.29D

anteriorly. Perpendicularity is helped by directing the patient's gaze away from the probe (Figure 3.29). The echograms are labelled according to the clock hour at the centre of the beam, and also to the beam's antero-

posterior location. For example, a section labelled 12 posterior (12P) is produced by a probe located at 6 o'clock limbus (Figure 3.29), a 6 equator (6E) by a probe located at 12 o'clock, mid-distance between lim-

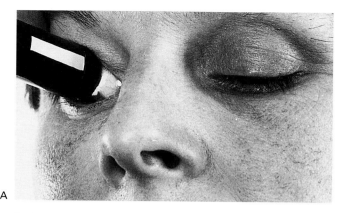

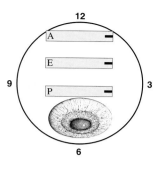

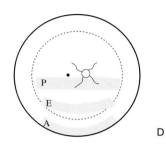

A

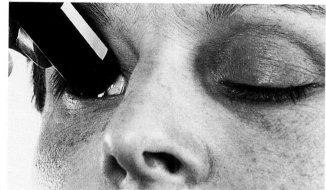

B

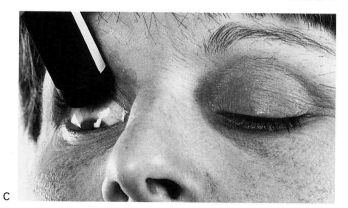

D

Figure 3.30 Transverse-6 B-scanning of right eye. Figures 3.30A, 3.30B, and 3.30C illustrate the direction of gaze and probe angle and position for sections 6P, 6E, and 6A respectively. As is conventional, the marker is located nasally. The concept is also presented in Figure 3.30D. The resulting echograms would be similar to those in Figure 3.29

C

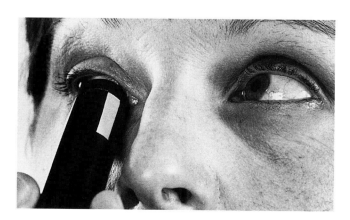

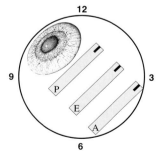

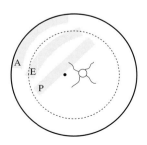

Figure 3.31 Transverse-10 B-scanning of right eye. In this instance the beam is centred at 10 o'clock, scanning the supra-temporal fundus

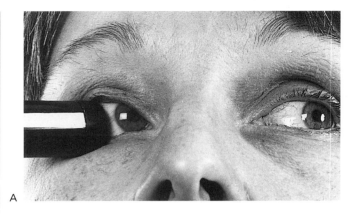

A

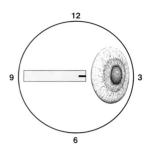

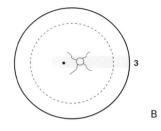

B

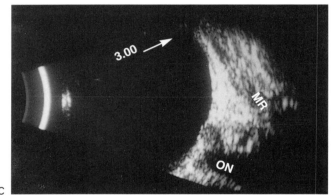

C

3.00 →

MR

ON

Figure 3.32 Longitudinal-3 B-scan of right eye. In Figure 3.32A, the patient directs the gaze at 3 o'clock and the probe is placed temporally with its marker towards the limbus. Figure 3.32B is a diagrammatic illustration of the probe's position on the globe and the beam orientation on the fundus. Figure 3.32C shows the actual echogram. The arrow points at the fundus periphery at 3 o'clock. ON = optic nerve, MR = long section of medial rectus

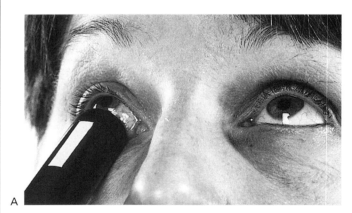

A

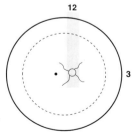

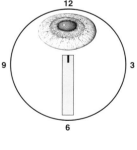

B

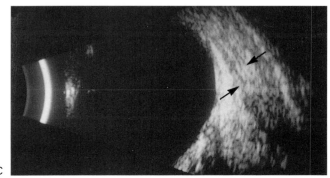

C

Figure 3.33 Longitudinal-12 scan of right eye. Figure 3.33A shows the patient's gaze and probe/marker position. Figure 3.33B is a schematic drawing of the probe's position on the eye and beam orientation on the fundus. Figure 3.33C is the resulting echogram. The superior rectus/levator complex is now displayed (two arrows), and the optic nerve is seen in its usual position at the bottom

bus and fornix (Figure 3.30), and a 10 anterior (10A) by a probe at 4 o'clock fornix (Figure 3.31). Note that in transverse sections it is conventional to orient the marker nasally instead of temporally, and superiorly instead of inferiorly.

Transverse sections provide information on the lateral extent of lesions and, by avoiding the lens, yield better resolution.

3. Longitudinal section

This section produces an antero-posterior slice of the ocular wall along one meridian only; from the optic nerve (lower portion of the echogram) to the ciliary body (upper portion of the echogram). The probe, therefore, is located on the sclera with the marker at its limbal side. The periphery and ciliary body are brought into view by directing the patient's gaze away from the probe, i.e. towards the meridian to be scanned. The echograms are labelled after the clock-hour location of the beam; for example, L-3 is a section produced by a probe at 9 o'clock limbus (Figure 3.32) and L-12 by a probe at 6 o'clock limbus (Figure 3.33).

Longitudinal scans are suitable for displaying the antero-posterior limits of lesions and the attachment of membranes to the optic nerve head.

Steps of ocular screening

A consistent routine is recommended. This comprises scanning the entire globe with four or eight overlapping transverse sections as follows (Figure 3.34A and B):

1. Transverse 12. The patient directs gaze superiorly. The probe is placed at the 6 o'clock limbus with its marker nasally. Shifting and rotating the probe from limbus to fornix scans the superior retina postero-anteriorly.
2. Transverse 3. The patient gazes at 3 o'clock and the probe is placed at 9 o'clock with its marker up. The probe is manoeuvred from limbus to fornix, scanning the nasal retina in the right eye and temporal retina in the left.
3. Transverse 6. The patient looks downwards and the probe is positioned at 12 o'clock, with the marker nasally, and swept from limbus to fornix to scan the inferior retina. If the superior orbital rim is prominent, scanning through the upper eyelid may facilitate visualization of the extreme periphery of the fundus.
4. Transverse 9. The patient gazes at 9 o'clock and the probe is manoeuvred at 3 o'clock, with its marker

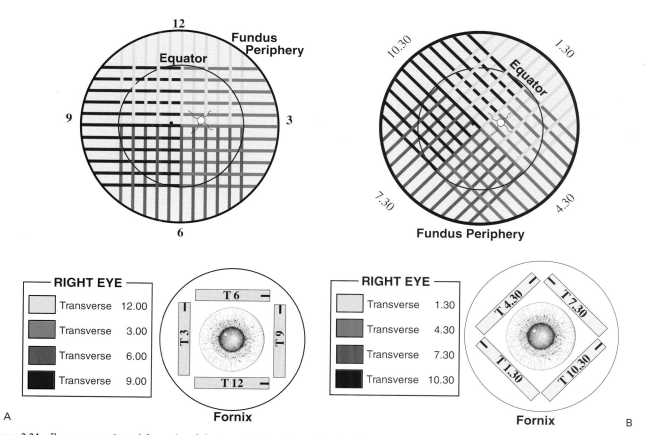

Figure 3.34 B-scan screening of the entire globe is undertaken by performing four overlapping transverse sections at 12, 3, 6, and 9 (Figure 3.34A), and an additional four sections centred at 1.30, 4.30, 7.30, and 10.30 clock hours (Figure 3.34B). Note that each quadrant of the fundus wall is scanned twice postero-anteriorly

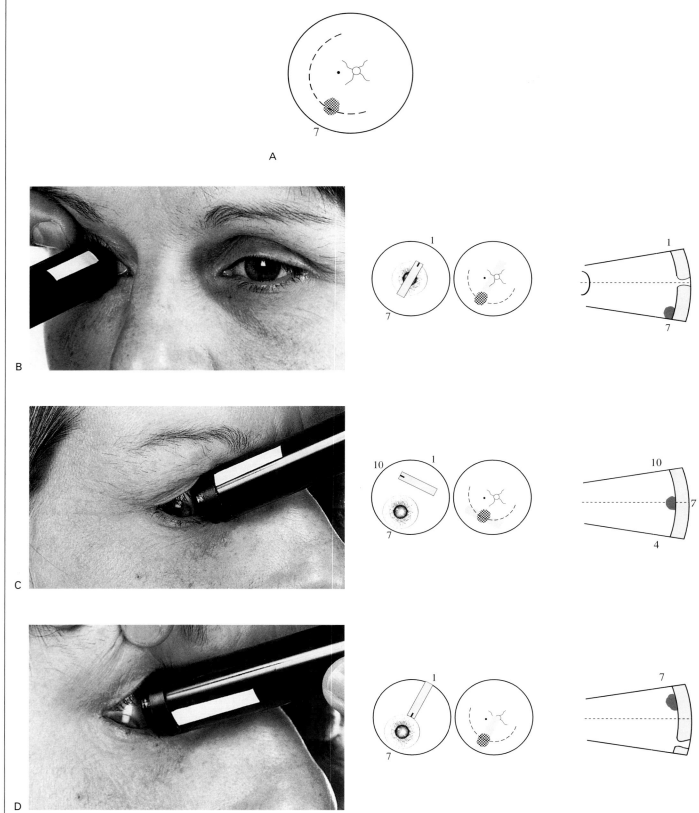

Figure 3.35 An example in the detection and localization of a lesion located at 7 o'clock equator, right eye (Figure 3.35A). The sections required for optimum display of the lesion are axial 1.00 (Figure 3.35B), transverse 7.00 (Figure 3.35C), and longitudinal 7.00 (Figure 3.35D). Illustrated are the location of probe and marker, the direction of gaze and beam projection on the fundus

kept up. This section scans the temporal retina in the right eye and nasal retina in the left.

5. Four additional transverse scans of the oblique quadrants – i.e. 1.30, 4.30, 7.30, and 10.30 clock hours – may be performed in a similar fashion (Figure 3.34B) if abnormalities in the oblique periphery are suspected.

Scans are performed first with a high decibel gain to detect fine vitreous opacities and thin detached posterior vitreous face, then repeated with a lower gain to examine layers of the ocular wall, the thickness of mass lesions, configurations of membranous opacities, etc.

If no lesion is found, no further examination is required. If a lesion is detected, longitudinal and axial sections are also performed. Multiple sections are helpful for viewing lesions from many angles, locating their meridian and antero-posterior position, and creating a three-dimensional impression. An example is illustrated in Figure 3.35.

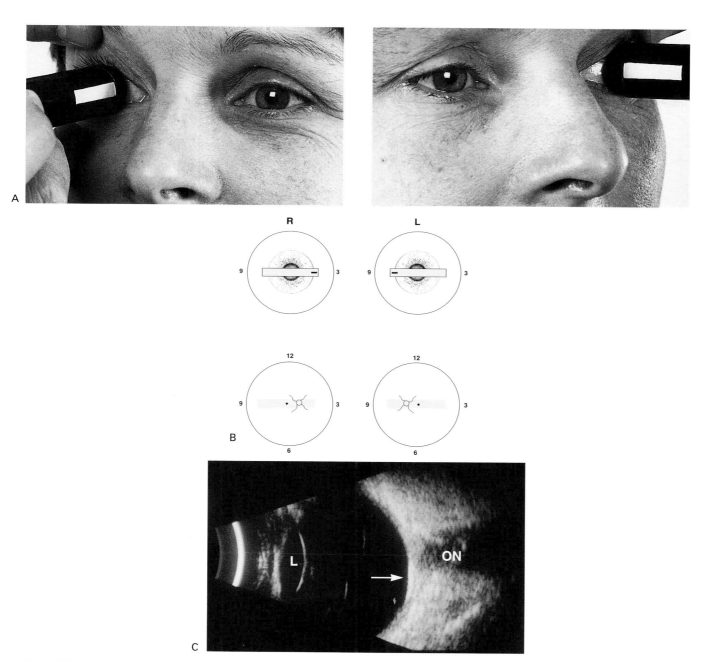

Figure 3.36   Axial macular screening. Figure 3.36A shows the eye and probe position (right and left). Figure 3.36B is a schematic drawing of probe and beam orientation. Note that the marker is located nasally in both eyes. Figure 3.36C shows the actual echogram. The macula (arrow) is displayed below the optic nerve (ON); L = lens

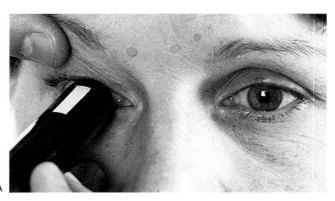

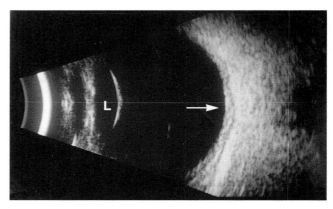

A   B

Figure 3.37   Vertical macula B-scan section. In Figure 3.37A the probe is placed on the central cornea with its marker up. Figure 3.37B is the actual echogram. L = lens; the arrow points at the macula

Macular screening

The macula can be screened via four approaches.

1. Horizontal axial (Figures 3.26, 3.36): An axial section with the marker nasally will display the macular area and adjacent optic nerve head. The familiar landmarks of lens and optic nerve allow easy-to-read echograms.
2. Vertical macula (Figure 3.37): A vertical axial section is first produced. The probe is then tilted temporally without losing the posterior lens echoes. The vertical beam is therefore shifted from the optic nerve to the macular area. The lens acts as a reference point for accurate placement of the beam and for future comparison.
3. Transverse 9.00 right eye and 3.00 left eye (Figure 3.38): The probe is placed on the corresponding nasal limbus with its marker up, and the patient gazes temporally. Avoiding the lens allows better visualization of the vertical extent of macular masses.
4. Longitudinal 9.00 right eye and 3.00 left eye (Figure 3.39): The patient's gaze is directed temporally. The probe is positioned on the nasal side of the globe with the marker at the limbus. The macular area will appear at the centre of the echogram, with the optic nerve at the bottom and the ciliary body at the top. The lateral extension of macular lesions is studied in this section.

Scanning of fundus periphery and ciliary body

This is aided by directing the patient's gaze maximally towards the meridian to be examined and applying a large quantity of coupling jelly to maintain good contact with the globe. Transverse and longitudinal sections of the periphery are produced by scanning from the opposite fornix (Figure 3.40).

Ciliary body masses can also be scanned by placing the probe directly over the lesion. In these cases, the tumour echoes are displayed immediately after the initial signal (Figure 3.41).

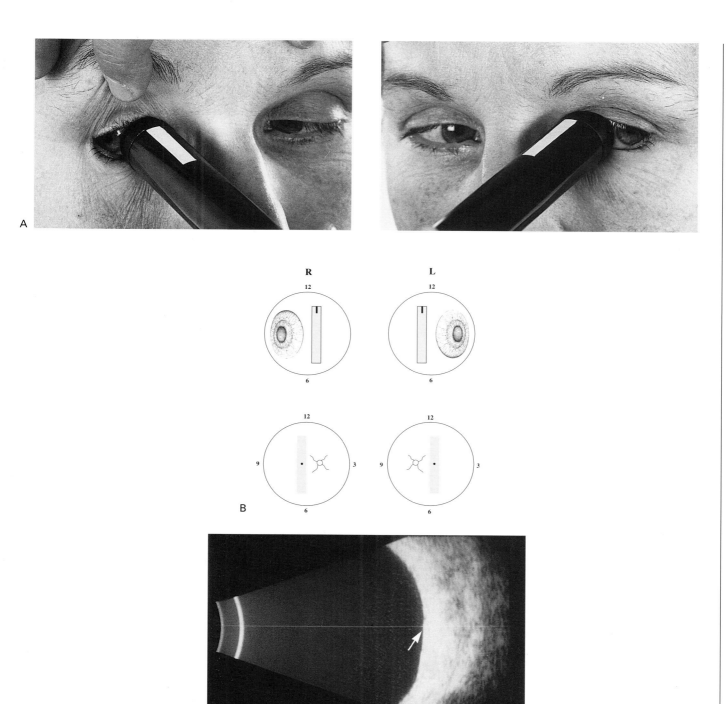

Figure 3.38 Transverse macular screening. Figures 3.38A and B illustrate the probe/eye position and the orientation of the beam on the fundus. Figure 3.38C is the resultant echogram. The macula is centred in the echogram for maximum resolution (arrow)

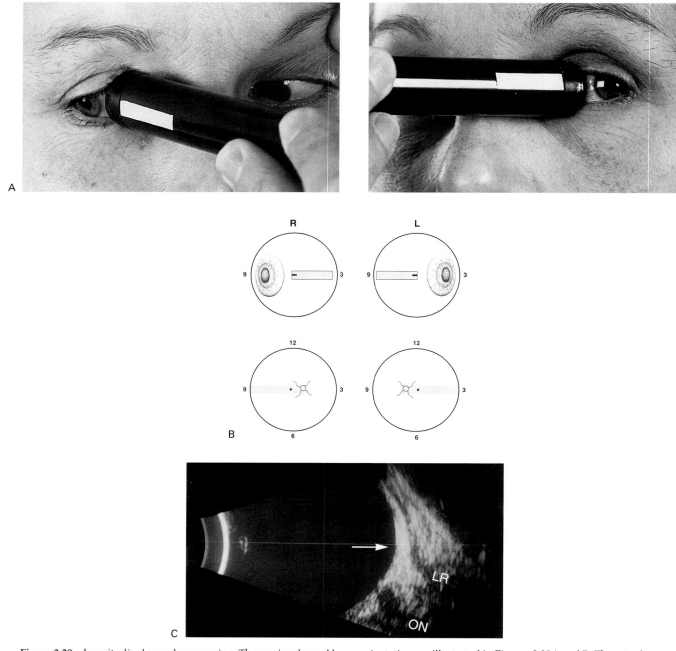

Figure 3.39 Longitudinal macular screening. The eye/probe and beam orientation are illustrated in Figures 3.39A and B. The actual echogram is shown in Figure 3.39C; the arrow points at the macula. As in all longitudinal sections, the optic nerve shadow appears at the bottom of the echogram (ON). The long section of the lateral rectus is also displayed (LR)

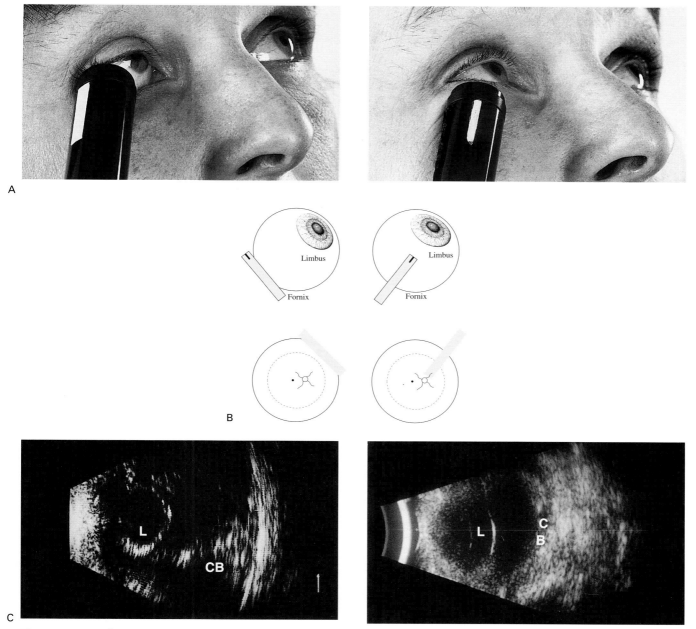

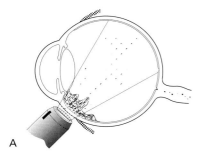

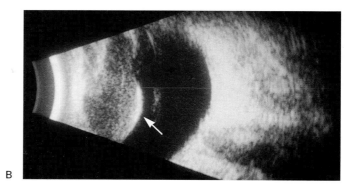

Figure 3.40 Peripheral globe and ciliary body screening. In Figure 3.40A, the probe is placed at the extreme fornix (left) or even on the lid skin (right) to help probe angling. Figure 3.40B is a diagrammatic illustration of probe/eye and beam orientation. Figure 3.40C shows the actual echograms. A tangential view of the lens (curved line L) and ciliary body (CB) is displayed.

Figure 3.41 Direct ciliary body B-scanning. In Figure 3.41A, the probe is placed on the sclera directly over the lesion. In Figure 3.41B, a ciliary body lesion (melanoma) is displayed to the left of the echogram (arrow)

IMMERSION SCANNING

The development of high-resolution, real-time contact B-scanners with their small, easy-to-manoeuvre probes has greatly reduced the need for immersion scanning.

A 'stand-off' technique is occasionally needed, however, in order to clearly display lesions in the anterior chamber, iris, ciliary body, and lens. This method may also be used when a very precise measurement of the anterior chamber depth, lens thickness, and globe axial length is required – e.g. during research studies – since it avoids corneal indentation.

Many implements for immersing the eye in a water bath have been devised. The best, however, are those allowing easy examination through the open eyelids, with the minimum of discomfort for the patient. One such device, originally produced by Hanson Ophthalmic Development Laboratories, Iowa City, comprises a set of cylindrical 'scleral shells' with a diameter of between 16 and 24 mm in width (Figure 3.42). One end of the shell is shelved to ensure a 'watertight' fit under the eyelids. After a topical anaesthetic has been applied, the shell is placed on the eye and filled with coupling jelly, care being taken to avoid trapping small air bubbles, which produce numerous artefacts. If the shell is properly fitted, saline solution is a better alternative to ultrasound gel in eliminating this problem (Figure 3.43).

Both A- and B-modes can be used in immersion scanning. The patient is first positioned with the face horizontal to avoid spillage of fluid, and the probe is placed on the fitted shell (Figure 3.44). In a normal axial scan, the echoes of the anterior and posterior corneal surfaces, iris and anterior lens (usually indistinguishable), and posterior lens can all be identified (Figure 3.45). A slight tilt and shift of the probe and shell will display the iris root and ciliary body.

Figures 3.46, 3.47, and 3.48 show examples of the possible range of lesions detectable by the immersion technique.

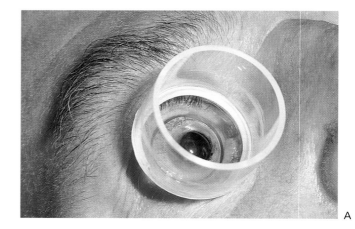

A

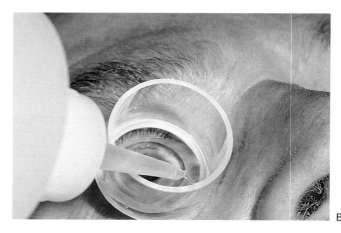

B

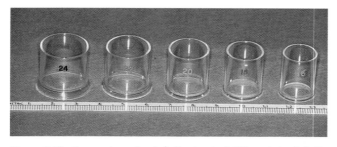

Figure 3.42 Immersion scleral shells. A set of different sized shells are supplied to ensure a 'watertight' fit. The shells illustrated are those originally produced by Hanson Ophthalmic Development Laboratories Co., Iowa City, USA

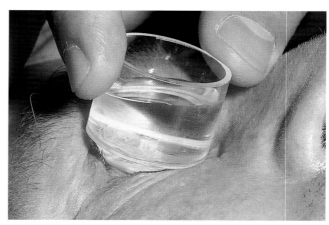

C

Figure 3.43 Application of immersion shell. In Figure 3.43A the shell is secured under the eyelids. In Figure 3.43B saline is introduced gently along the shell wall. In Figure 3.43C, the shell is three-quarters filled with saline. The patient's head and the shell are adjusted to maintain a horizontal fluid level

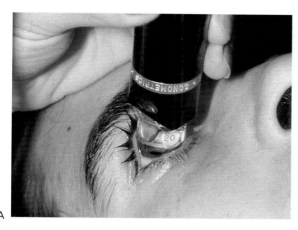
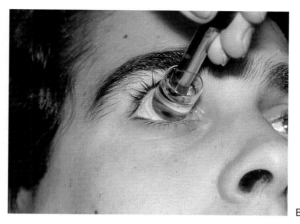

Figure 3.44 B- and A-scan probes (Figures 3.44A and 3.44B) are placed in contact with the fluid level in the shell. (Courtesy of SF Byrne)

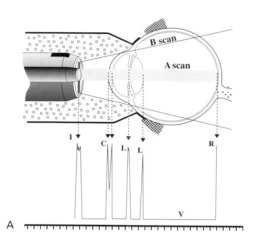

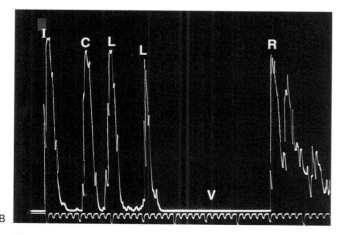
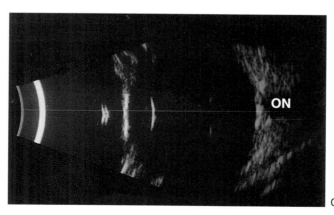

Figure 3.45 Immersion ultrasound. Both A- and B-scans can be utilized. The usual anatomical landmarks in the normal eye are illustrated (Figure 3.45A). I = initial spike, C = corneal spikes (anterior and posterior), L = anterior lens/iris and posterior lens spikes, V = vitreous, R = retina, ON = optic nerve. The echogram for A-scan is shown in Figure 3.45B, and for B-scan in Figure 3.45C

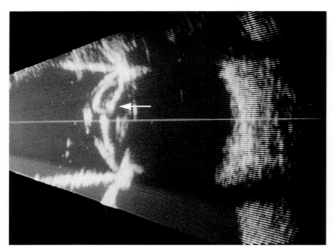

Figure 3.46 A vertical immersion B-scan of a superior iris cyst (arrow)

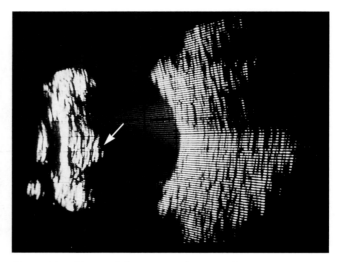

Figure 3.47 Traumatic lens rupture/cataract. Immersion scan showing high echoes in the lens, indicating cataract, and an irregular posterior lens surface (arrow) (cf. Figure 3.45C) (courtesy of S.F. Byrne)

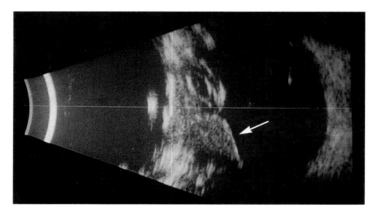

Figure 3.48 An immersion scan of a large inferior ciliary body melanoma (arrow). The lesion is seen pushing and subluxating a cataractous lens above it

REFERENCES

1 Ossoinig K C. Basics of echographic tissue differentiation, II: Acoustic behaviour of biological structures. In: Boeck J, Ossoinig K C (eds) Ultrasonographia medica. Vienna: Verlag Wiener Med. Akademie, 1971:419–439 (In German)

2 Ossoinig K C. Basics of echographic tissue differentiation, I: Experimental and clinical examinations of the influence of system parameters on the diagnostic value of echograms. In: Boeck J, Ossoinig K C (eds) Ultrasonographia medica. Vienna: Verlag Wiener Med. Akademie, 1971:155–168 (In German)

3 Ossoinig K C. The first standardized system for echo-ophthalmolography. In: Massin, Poujol J (eds) Diagnostica ultrasonica in ophthalmologia (Proceedings of the SIDUO IV, Paris 1971). Paris: Centre National d'Ophthalmologie des Quinze-Vingts, 1973: 131–137 (In German)

4 Ossoinig K C, Patel J H. A-scan instrumentation for acoustic tissue differentiation, II: Clinical significance of various technical parameters of the 7200 MA unit of Kretztechnik. In: White D, Brown R E (eds) Ultrasound in medicine, Vol 3B. New York: Plenum, 1977; 1949–1954

5 Ossoinig K C. Standardized Echography: basic principles, clinical applications, and results. Int Ophthalmol Clinics 1979; 19:127–210

6 Ossoinig K C. The significance of the S-shaped amplifier characteristics in echographic tissue diagnosis. Doc Ophthalmol Proc Series 1981; 29:441–443

7 Till P. Solid tissue model for the standardization of the echo-ophthalmograph 7200 MA (Kretztechnik). Doc Ophthalmol. 1976; 41:205

8 Till P, Ossoinig K C. First experience with a new tissue model for the standardization of A- and B-scan instruments used in tissue diagnosis. In: White D, Brown R E (eds) Ultrasound in medicine, Vol 3B. New York: Plenum, 1977:2167–2174.

4

Special examination techniques: globe

In the previous chapter a methodical approach to screening of the globe with A- and B-scan was described, with the advantage that a consistent routine will be developed, thus ensuring a high detection rate and meaningful follow-up studies.

In this chapter the special examination techniques required to reach an echographic diagnosis are discussed, namely topographic, kinetic, and quantitative echography. Table 2.1 summarizes these techniques, the acoustic information they provide and the scanning mode best used to obtain them.

TOPOGRAPHIC EXAMINATION

This involves the assessment of shape, extension, location, and other 'qualitative' features of the lesion. In the eye this is usually performed with B-scan, supplemented by A-scan.

Abnormal topographic findings in the globe can be classified into four major groups:

1. Mass lesion (Figure 4.1).
2. Membranous opacity (Figure 4.2).
3. Discrete (single or multiple) vitreous opacities (Figure 4.3).
4. Abnormalities in globe contour (Figure 4.4).

A mass lesion can be described, if mild, as thickening of the chorio-retinal layer, dome-shaped, 'bi-domed', mushroom, conical, or irregularly shaped.

Topographic evaluation of membranous opacities includes their attachment to the optic nerve head, their extent and configuration – e.g. open or closed funnel – and their angle of insertion into the globe wall. The presence of folds, breaks, cysts, and cords in relation to the membrane is helpful in determining the nature of the opacity.

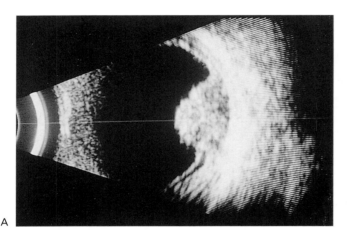

A

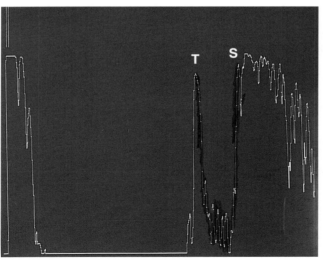

B

Figure 4.1 An example of a 'solid mass' ocular opacity (choroidal melanoma). Figure 4.1A: the B-scan showing a dome-shaped, bright mass, originating from the fundus. Figure 4.1B: an A-scan. The lesion's internal spikes between T (tumour surface spike) and S (scleral signal) can be described as medium low reflective, regularly structured with moderate sound attenuation. These features are characteristic of choroidal melanoma

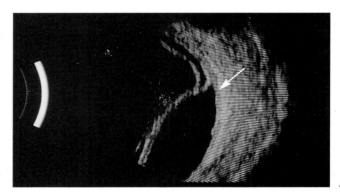

A

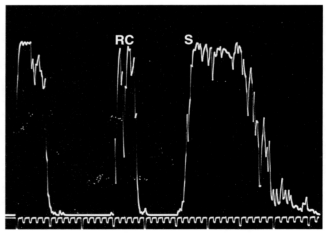

B

Figure 4.2 An example of a 'membranous' ocular opacity (choroidal effusion). Figure 4.2A: a B-scan showing a smooth dome-shaped linear opacity, which splits into two lines (retina and choroid) as it merges with the ocular wall (arrow). The dark (echo-silent) space between the linear opacity and the ocular wall indicates the 'non-solid' nature of the lesion. Figure 4.2B: the A-scan, showing a double-peaked, thick spike produced by the retina (R) and choroid (C). The space between the choroid (C) and sclera (S) contains no spikes, indicating a clear fluid (effusion) rather than haemorrhage in the supra-choroidal space

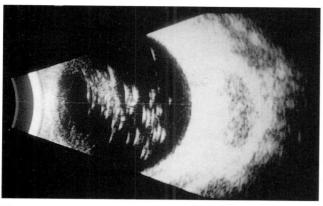
A

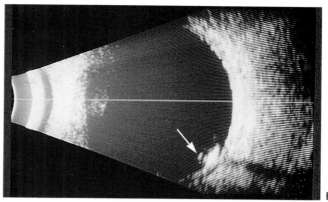
B

Figure 4.3 Examples of 'discrete' ocular opacities, multiple in Figure 4.3A and single in Figure 4.3B. In Figure 4.3A, the classical B-scan appearance of asteroid hyalosis is demonstrated. Note the clear vitreous zone before the ocular wall, indicating a shallow posterior vitreous detachment, commonly seen with this condition. In Figure 4.3B a single high-reflective foreign-body opacity is seen adjacent to the globe wall (arrow), producing the characteristic shadowing effect

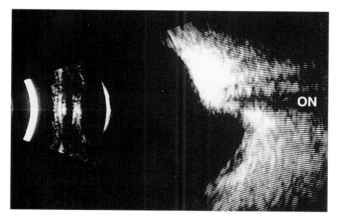

Figure 4.4 An example of abnormal globe wall contour: this vertical axial B-scan shows a marked pouching (posterior staphyloma) below the optic nerve (ON). The upper segment of the posterior globe wall is relatively normal

The size, density, and location of vitreous opacities are examined, and their relation to the posterior vitreous face and globe wall is determined.

Abnormalities of the globe contour include extremes of axial length, flattening, or pouching (staphyloma). In such cases comparison with the other eye is essential.

Once a lesion has been detected following the initial screening, precise orientation of its antero-posterior and meridian position is undertaken by performing transverse, longitudinal, and axial sections as described in Chapter 3. This will also determine the antero-posterior and lateral configuration. Figure 4.5 provides an exercise in the topographic evaluation of a solid mass in the right eye located in the 11 o'clock equator and associated with a supero-temporal retinal detachment.

Figure 4.5 An exercise in the topographic evaluation of a lesion in the supra-temporal quadrant of the right eye. In Figure 4.5A, the lesion is detected during initial B-scan screening on the T-12E and T-9E sections. Note that the lesion is located at the periphery (least sensitive) portion of the echograms. In order to centre the lesion in the echogram and locate its exact position, transverse (T-11E) and longitudinal (L-11) sections should be carried out, as shown in Figure 4.5B

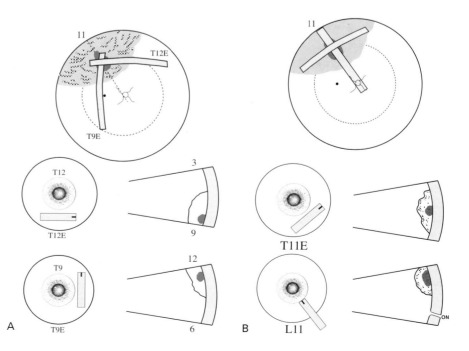

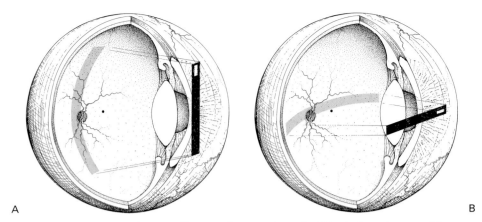

A   B

Figure 4.6   Kinetic evaluation of lesions. This is performed within the lateral sweep of the B-scan beam. In Figure 4.6A (vertical axial), the patient would be asked to look up and down, while in Figure 4.6B (horizontal axial) the eye movement would be in a horizontal direction, so that in both cases the movements of lesions are visible at all times

KINETIC ECHOGRAPHY

The dynamic examination of normal and abnormal ocular structures is an invaluable component of the echographic investigation. Both A- and B-scans can provide the following kinetic data:

1. Tissue mobility

The best example is that of the unique, freely undulating, 'hammock-like' motility of the vitreous body and posterior vitreous detachment versus the steady, 'curtain-like' movement of retinal detachment; both are associated with eye movements. B-scan is best suited for demonstrating the kinetics of membranes during eye movements. This is performed by asking the patient to rotate the eye back and forth within the lateral extension of the sound beam (Figure 4.6). This is important in enabling the examiner constantly to observe the image – otherwise the area of interest will 'come in and out' of view as the eye is rotated in and out of the beam path. A-scan, on the other hand, is more sensitive in demonstrating 'after-movements', i.e. the inertia of membranes immediately after the cessation of eye movements. Vitreous spikes tend to freely oscillate vertically and shift laterally along the base line, while the spike of retinal detachment exhibits fewer vertical, 'spring-like' vibrations and minimum lateral shift (Figure 4.7). Although it is difficult to illustrate on a still photograph, Figure 4.8 captures the excessive motility of synchysis scintillans.

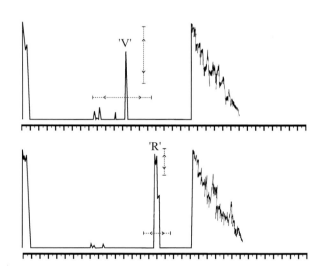

Figure 4.7   Kinetic A-scan assessment of membrane spikes (after-movement). The vertical oscillation and lateral shift are observed while the probe is kept still on the eye. The vitreous spike V (top) produces excessive vertical and lateral movements. The retinal signal R (bottom) produces limited, spring-like, vertical oscillations and minimal lateral shift

2. Vascularity

This is a significant finding in the assessment of intraocular tumours. Vascularity is normally detected on A-scan by the fine, fast, vertical vibration of internal tumour spikes, observed while the probe and patient's gaze are kept very still (Figure 4.9). When marked, it can also be seen on B-scan. Modern Doppler instruments have been successfully employed to demonstrate the vasculature of intraocular tumours.[1] Vascularity is considered a characteristic feature of malignant melanoma (Figure 4.10), as it is less commonly seen in metastatic disease and other intraocular lesions.[2,3,4]

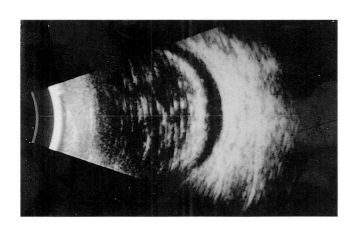

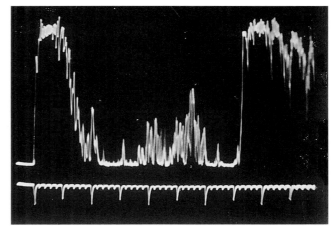

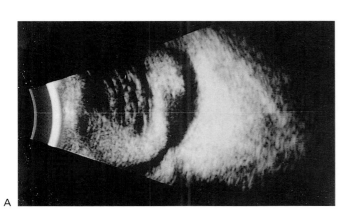

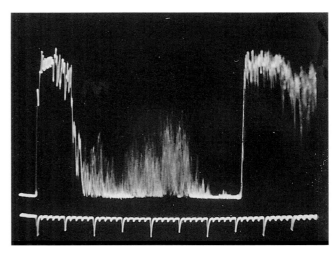

A

B

Figure 4.8 Kinetic echography of synchysis scintillans. Figure 4.8A: Transverse (top) and longitudinal (bottom) B-scans showing dense, dispersed vitreous opacities, maximally seen near the detached posterior hyaloid. Figure 4.8B: The A-scan traces are photographed before (top) and immediately following (bottom) a burst of saccadic eye movements. The blurred image of the synchysis spikes is clearly seen in the bottom echogram, indicating excessive motility

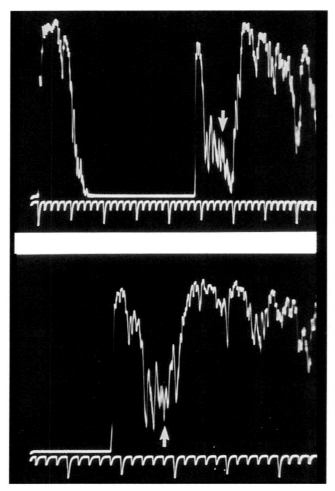

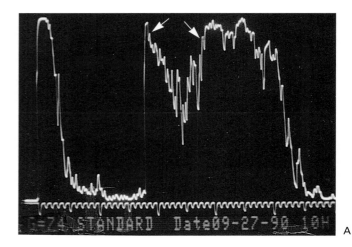

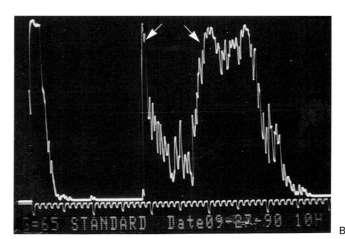

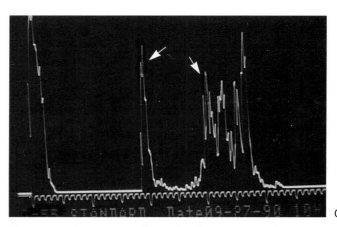

Figure 4.9 Kinetic echography of vascular tumours. Two A-scan echograms of choroidal melanoma demonstrating 'internal vascularity'. This is detected from the fast vertical oscillation of some spikes within the tumour; these appear on the still photograph as blurred, indistinct spikes (arrows) (Courtesy of S F Byrne)

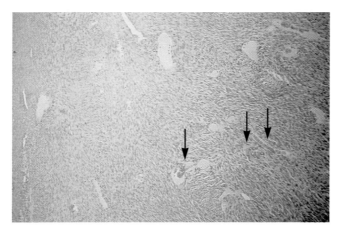

Figure 4.10 'A-scan' vascularity of melanomas is considered diagnostic. The focal vascular pattern seen on this histological section (arrows) explains the A-scan appearance of vascularity, described in Figure 4.9. Marked vascularity may also be detected during B-scan examination

Figure 4.11 Quantitative echography: the importance of setting T-sensitivity. These three A-scan traces are taken from the same area of a choroidal melanoma. Figure 4.11A is a T + 9 gain, Figure 4.11B a T-sensitivity gain, and Figure 4.11C a T − 10 gain. Note the marked change of appearance of the tumour (spikes between arrows). Only the T-sensitivity trace (Figure 4.11B) shows the recognisable features of melanoma

QUANTITATIVE ECHOGRAPHY

While B-scan supplies 'semi-quantitative' information on the intensity of echo-sources, A-scan is a more objective and precise method for obtaining data on reflectivity, internal structure, and sound attenuation of tissues. The need for 'standardization' of equipments (amplification and T-sensitivity) and examination techniques (perpendicularity) is self-evident if accurate and reliable measurements are to be taken of such parameters (Figure 4.11).

Reflectivity is the measurement of height (amplitude) of spikes. This can be an absolute value in decibels or a percentage comparison between the initial spike (100% tall) and the spike in question (Figure 4.12). The sclera, being the most highly reflective structure in the ocular wall, can also be used as a 'biological' reference for other tissues, particularly retinal detachment and posterior vitreous detachment (see p. 54, Figure 4.38).

Internal structure describes the regularity of spikes in terms of their height and interval. Regularly structured spikes tend to originate from regular (small or large) histological 'units', giving rise to homogeneous acoustic interfaces, e.g. choroidal melanoma and choroidal haemangioma. The opposite applies to irregularly structured lesions such as choroidal metastasis and disciform macular scar (Figure 4.13).

Sound attenuation is the angle of decline of spikes' height (angle kappa) along the beam path, produced by sound absorption. Normally, highly reflective, regularly structured lesions with small acoustic interfaces produce the strongest sound absorption and consequently the steepest decline in spikes' height.

The application of the special examination techniques is best illustrated by the description of two common groups of ocular abnormalities, membranous opacities and intraocular tumours.

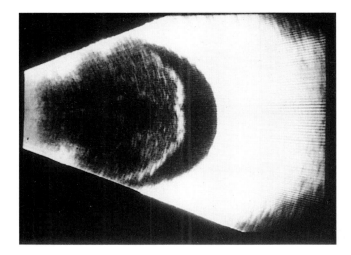

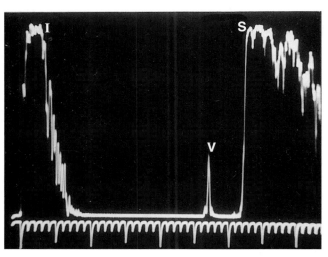

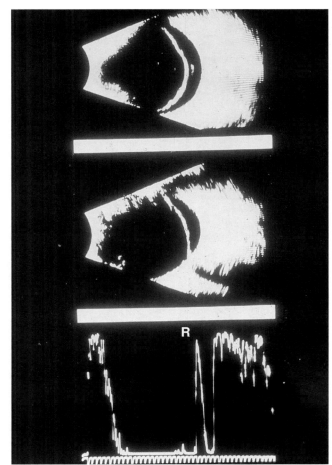

Figure 4.12 Quantiative echography of intraocular membranes. Figure 4.12A shows a transverse B-scan (top) and T-sensitivity A-scan (bottom) of posterior vitreous detachment (PVD). The B-scan shows fine dispersed vitreous opacities. Note the height of PVD spike (V) on the A-scan; this measures 30% of the initial spike (I) or sclera (S). Figure 4.12B shows a transverse and longitudinal B-scan (top and middle) and T-sensitivity A-scan (bottom) of retinal detachment. The height of the retinal spike (arrow) is almost 100%

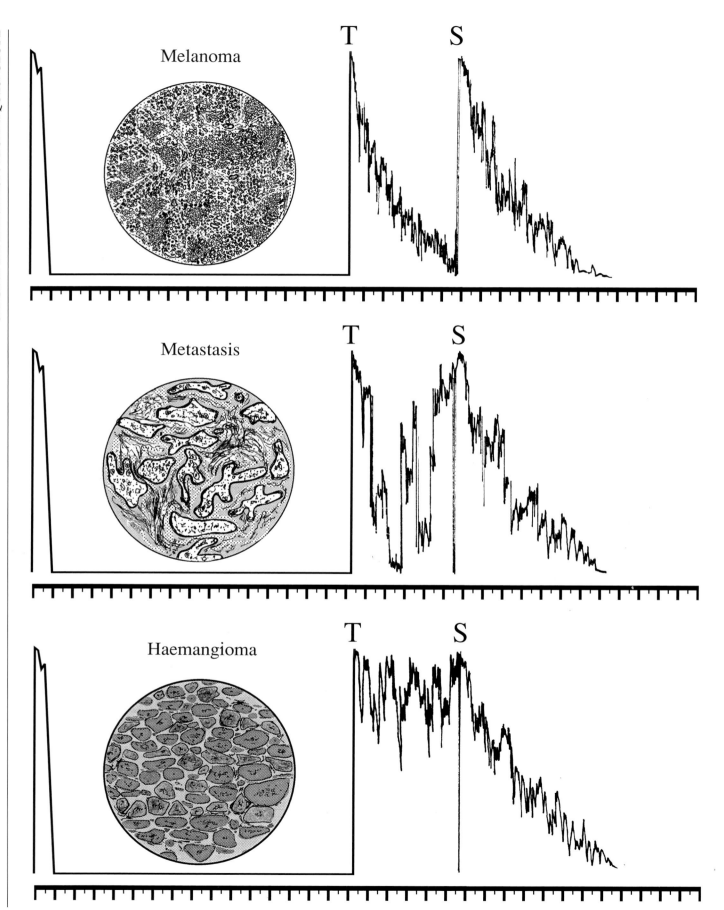

Figure 4.13 Quantitative A-scan echography of intraocular masses. The appearance of melanoma, metastasis, and choroidal haemangioma in relation to their histological architecture is diagrammatically presented. In melanoma, the small, tightly packed cells produce regular, small 'echographic interfaces', which in turn give rise to homogeneous (regular) internal structure, low to medium reflectivity, and significant sound attenuation. Metastasis usually has an irregular histological architecture (depending on the primary tumour), resulting in an irregular internal structure with variable reflectivity and sound attenuation. Choroidal haemangioma is regular but with large (honeycomb) spaces producing large echographic interfaces, its A-scan appearance is consistent with a regularly structured, highly reflective lesion with minimal sound attenuation.
T = tumour surface spike. S = scleral signal

MEMBRANOUS OPACITIES

Three membranous opacities are commonly encountered during ultrasound examination: choroidal detachment, retinal detachment, and posterior vitreous detachment.

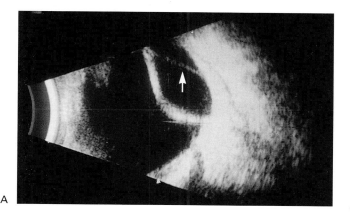

A

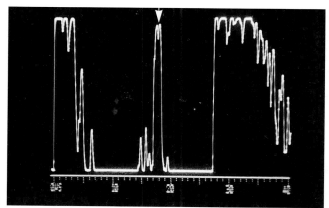

B

Figure 4.14 Choroidal detachment (effusion). Figure 4.14A is a longitudinal B-scan. The detached choroid appears as a thick, bright, dome-shaped opacity inserting abruptly into the globe wall, anterior to the optic nerve. The supra-choroidal space is echo-silent, indicating clear effusion. A vortex vein (arrow) is also seen. Figure 4.14B is a T-sensitivity A-scan. The choroidal spike (arrow) is typically double-peaked and almost 100% tall

Choroidal detachment

On *topographic* evaluation, choroidal detachment appears as a smooth, dome-shaped lesion, occupying the fundus periphery and inserting abruptly into the globe wall (Figure 4.14). Two or more separate domes are frequently present and, if very high, they may touch in mid vitreous, producing the so-called 'kissing choroids' (Figure 4.15). In annular choroidal detachment, often associated with ciliary body detachment and hypotony, the choroid forms a continuous 360° shallow peripheral linear opacity (Figure 4.16). Very peripheral transverse B-scan sections are required in such cases. Choroidal detachments, however extensive, do not attach to the optic nerve head, a feature best verified on longitudinal sections (Figures 4.14A, 4.15B). Depending on the cause, the supra-choroidal space may be anechoic, as in choroidal effusion (Figure 4.14), or contain dispersed opacities, as in haemorrhagic detachment (Figure 4.17). Occasionally a linear, cord-like, thin opacity is seen stretching from the detached choroidal layer to the ocular wall (Figure 4.14). This is presumed to be a vortex vein. The base dimensions of the detachment are measured on transverse and longitudinal B-scan and the height on perpendicular A-scan sections using measuring (dB)

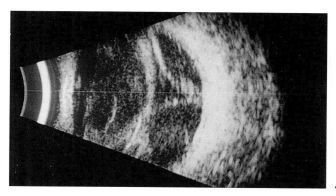

A

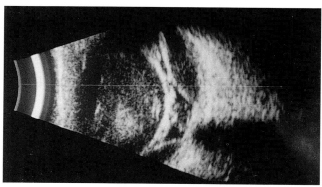

B

Figure 4.15 Choroidal detachment: 'kissing choroids' seen in a case of traumatic haemorrhagic choroidal detachment. Figure 4.15A is a transverse B-scan showing three high choroidal domes touching in mid-vitreous. Echoes in the supra-choroidal spaces indicate haemorrhage. Figure 4.15B is a longitudinal B-scan demonstrating the three 'kissing choroids' and showing that the membranes attach near, but not into, the optic nerve, excluding retinal detachment

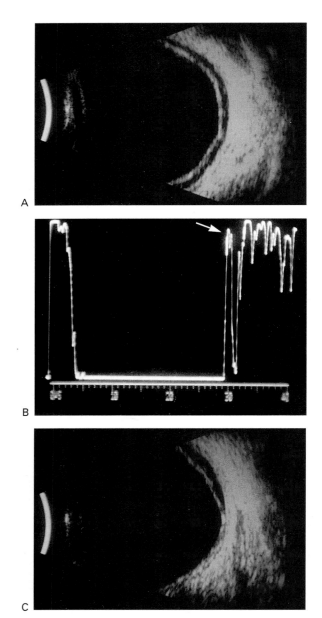

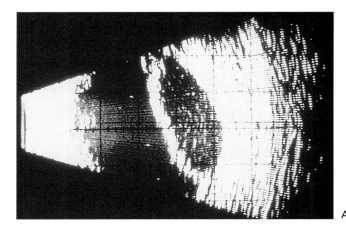

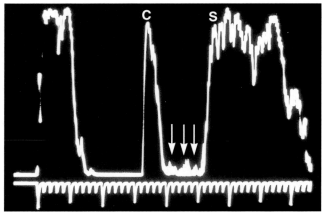

Figure 4.17 Haemorrhagic choroidal detachment. Figure 4.17A: B-scan showing fine, dispersed opacities in the supra-choroidal space, indicating haemorrhage. Figure 4.17B: A-scan, with haemorrhage represented by a chain of low reflective spikes (arrow) between the choroidal detachment (C) and sclera (S)

Figure 4.16 Annular choroidal detachment associated with chronic hypotony following trabeculectomy. Figure 4.16A: peripheral transverse B-scan showing shallow choroidal detachment running parallel to the globe wall, an appearance that was similar in all quadrants. Figure 4.16B: A-scan showing a high, thick choroidal signal (arrow) adjacent to the scleral spike. Figure 4.16C: longitudinal B-scan showing the detachment extending as far back as the equator

sensitivity (Figure 4.18). Measurements are helpful in assessing progression of the condition, particularly if fundoscopy is hampered.

In the *quantitative* examination, the choroid produces a thick, bright opacity on B-scan, even at low gain setting, and a thick, double-peaked, 90–100% tall spike on A-scan (Figure 4.14).

On *kinetic* echography, choroidal detachment produces minimum mobility and very slight or no after-movement.

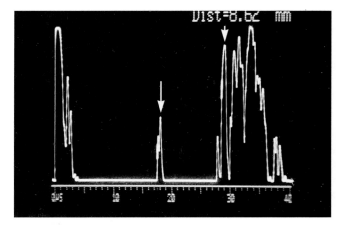

Figure 4.18 A-scan measurement of height of choroidal detachment. A perpendicular trace is first obtained at T sensitivity (100% tall, smooth choroidal and scleral spikes, as in Figure 4.14B). The sensitivity is lowered by 10 to 20 dB. The distance between the peaks of the two spikes (arrows) is measured. In the example illustrated, the height is 8.62 mm

Retinal detachment

In the *topographic* examination, retinal detachment appears as a membranous opacity. This may be smooth (Figure 4.19) or 'folded', the latter may indicate early proliferative vitreo-retinopathy (PVR) (Figure 4.20). The membrane normally separates gradually from the ocular wall (unlike in choroidal detachment) (Figure 4.19). Unless it is limited to the periphery, the opacity inserts into the optic nerve head (Figures 4.21, 4.22), a feature best seen on longitudinal B-scan sections. Careful B-scanning at low gain, especially of the upper periphery, may demonstrate a break, which, if found, indicates a large tear (Figure 4.23). Giant tears, which are common in Stickler's disease, can easily be seen with their rolled edges (Figure 4.24). Total retinal detachment produces a V-shaped opacity anchored to the optic nerve head. The angle of the 'V' varies depending on the degree of vitreo-retinal traction/adhesion (Figures 4.21, 4.22).

Other topographic features include peripheral retinal looping and cyst formation, frequently found in long-standing detachments (Figure 4.25). The sub-retinal space may contain fine dispersed opacities

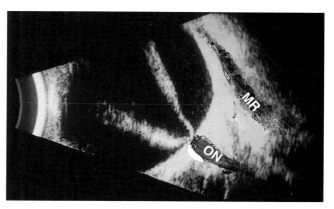

Figure 4.21 Longitudinal B-scan showing an open-funnel retinal detachment attached to the optic nerve. ON = optic nerve, MR = medial rectus muscle

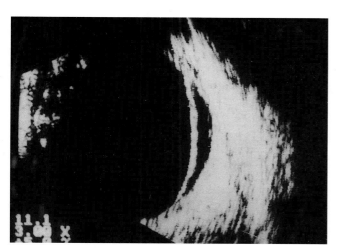

Figure 4.19 Shallow (early) retinal detachment, appearing as smooth, linear opacity, merging gradually with the globe wall

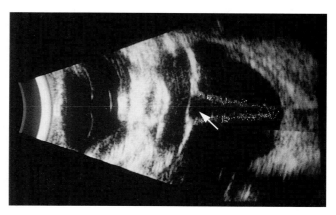

Figure 4.22 Closed or narrow-funnel retinal detachment, producing a 'table-top' appearance. The funnel is bridged by a membrane (arrow), indicating severe PVR

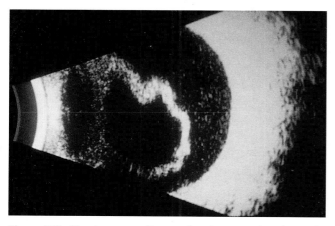

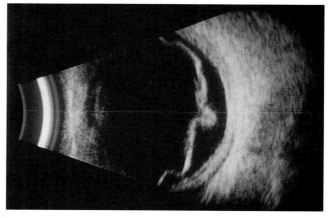

Figure 4.20 Two transverse B-scans showing examples of retinal detachments with the characteristic 'folds', indicating early stages of proliferative vitreo-retinopathy (PVR). The echogram to the left also shows fine, dispersed opacities (blood) in the subretinal space

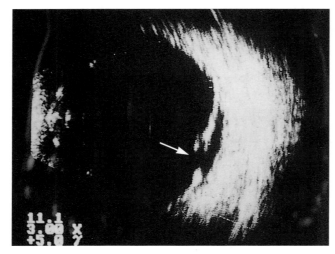

Figure 4.23 Peripheral transverse B-scan showing a retinal break (arrow) surrounded by a shallow retinal detachment

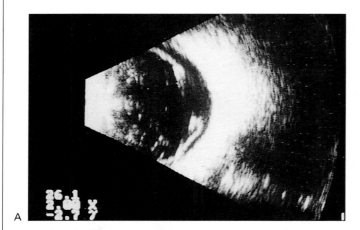

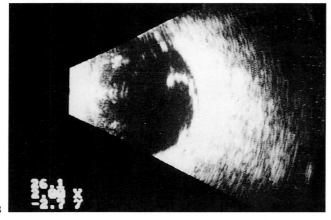

Figure 4.24 Transverse (Figure 4.24A) and longitudinal (Figure 4.24B) B-scans in a case of Stickler's disease. A giant tear with rolled edges is clearly demonstrated

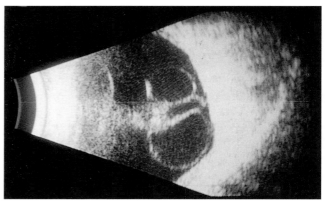

Figure 4.25 Long-standing, closed-funnel retinal detachment with two large subretinal cysts

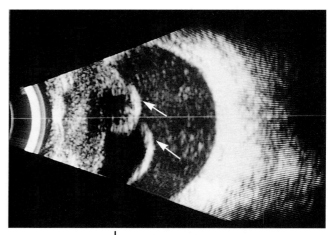

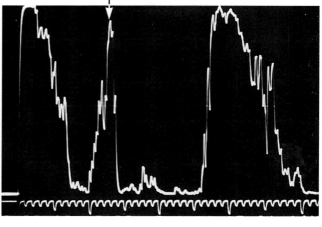

Figure 4.26 Transverse B-scan (Figure 4.26A) and A-scan (Figure 4.26B) of a case of advanced Coats' disease. The retina is totally detached (arrows) and the subretinal space contains coarse, dispersed (cholesterol) opacities. (Reproduced with permission from Atta H R, Watson N J. Echographic diagnosis of advanced Coats' disease. Eye 6:80–85 1992)

(fresh blood), commonly seen in diabetic patients (Figure 4.20), coarse scattered opacities, as in chronic or exudative detachments – the best example Coats' disease (Figure 4.26) – and taut 'cord-like' bands indicative of subretinal fibrosis (Figure 4.27).

Quantitative examination shows a bright, thick membrane on B-scan and a 90–100% tall spike on A-scan (Figure 4.28). Assessment of the A-scan reflectivity, however, can only be made accurately on perpendicular sections.[5] A weaker retinal signal, par-

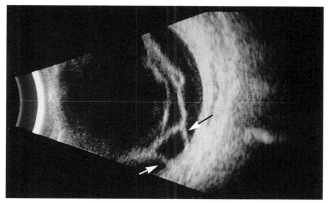

A

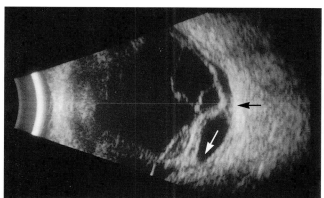

B

Figure 4.27 Two B-scans from a patient showing a complex web of long-standing retinal detachment, vitreo-retinal fibrosis, and subretinal cord opacities (arrows). Kinetic examination of this case showed very poor mobility of the retina

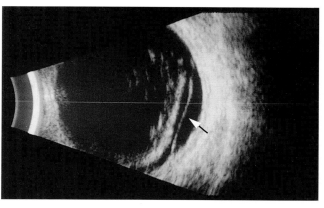

Figure 4.29 A case of localized retinal detachment, appearing as a thin, weakly reflective membrane (arrow) behind a zone of dense vitreous opacities (asteroid hyalosis), condensed near the detached posterior hyaloid. These findings were confirmed at vitrectomy

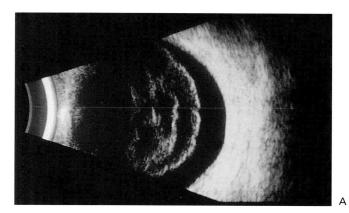

A

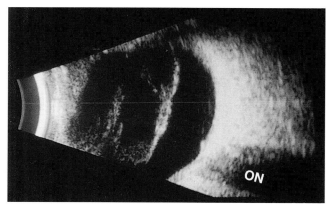

B

Figure 4.30 Posterior vitreous detachment (PVD). The posterior hyaloid face demarcates vitreous opacities (haemorrhage) from a clear retro-hyaloid space. The second membrane-like opacity in Figure 4.30A (arrow) indicates a degree of vitreous seneresis. The longitudinal section in Figure 4.30B shows no attachment of PVD to the optic nerve (ON)

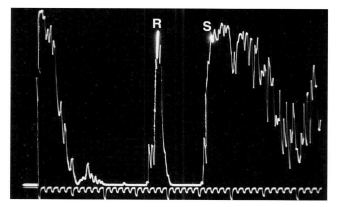

Figure 4.28 Quantitative A-scan of retinal detachment. This T-sensitivity scan with optimum (perpendicular) beam alignment shows the retina as a 100% tall spike (R), compared to the sclera (S)

ticularly on B-scan, is occasionally encountered if the vitreous cavity is heavily laden with dense opacities such as thick blood or asteroid hyalosis. This is probably due to the reduction of sound energy as it reaches the detached retina (Figure 4.29).

Kinetic echography illustrates a moderately mobile opacity on B-scan and a rapid inertia upon cessation of eye movement. The characteristic short vertical oscillation and limited lateral shift on A-scan (after-movements) are also observed (Figure 4.7).

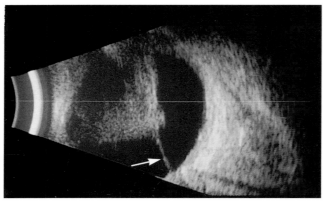

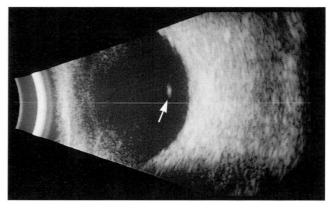

Figure 4.31 PVD attached to the optic nerve. Figure 4.31A: a longitudinal B-scan demonstrating a PVD anchored to the optic nerve by a thin linear opacity (arrow). Figure 4.31B: a transverse (cross-section) B-scan shows the linear opacity as a dot (arrow), confirming its cord-like structure

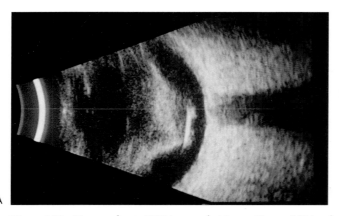

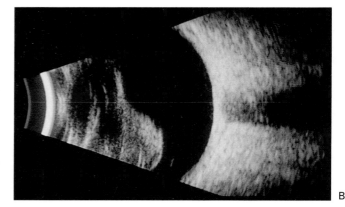

Figure 4.32 Haemorrhagic PVD in an aphakic eye. Figure 4.32A: a horizontal axial B-scan; the PVD is the same distance, nasally and temporally, from the globe wall. Figure 4.32B: vertical axial scan; the PVD is higher superiorly

Posterior vitreous detachment (PVD)

Topographic examination shows a linear, membranous opacity that may or may not attach to the optic nerve (Figures 4.30, 4.31). The distance of the membrane from the posterior ocular wall is normally greater at the upper quadrants (Figure 4.32). PVD can be complete or incomplete, with one or more areas of vitreo-retinal adhesions. This is commonly seen at the macula (as in cases of 'idiopathic' macular hole), at the vascular arcades (in patients with proliferative diabetic retinopathy (Figure 4.33) and old retinal vein occlusion (Figure 4.34)), and at the periphery (where a retinal tear should be suspected). Occasionally, the membrane demarcates intravitreous opacities from a clear retro-hyaloid space, except in cases where the PVD is associated with a haemorrhagic retinal break, or in diabetic retinopathy when fine dispersed echoes are also seen in the retro-hyaloid space (Figure 4.35).

Sometimes, the B-scan appearance of open-funnel retinal detachment and thick PVD attached to the optic nerve can be very similar, and invariably requires additional (A-scan) quantitative and kinetic information before the correct diagnosis can be reached.[6,7]

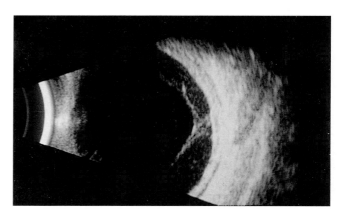

Figure 4.33 Incomplete PVD in proliferative diabetic retinopathy. Broad adhesion between the posterior hyaloid and retina, preventing total vitreous detachment, is seen. A mild degree of subhyaloid haemorrhage is also present. Vitreo-retinal adhesions are common in the pre-equatorial (vascular arcades) regions in eyes with diabetic retinopathy

On *quantitative* examination, PVD produces a much weaker, thinly peaked spike on A-scan, varying in height from 40 to 80% of the scleral signal (Figures 4.35, 4.36, 4.37). Even so, a thick PVD, especially inferiorly,

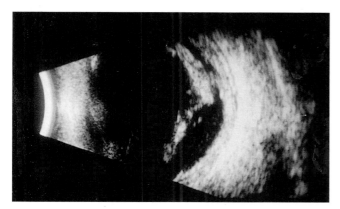

Figure 4.34 Incomplete 'haemorrhagic' PVD in an eye with a long-standing central retinal vein occlusion. Note the focal thickening of the chorio-retinal layer at the area of adhesion

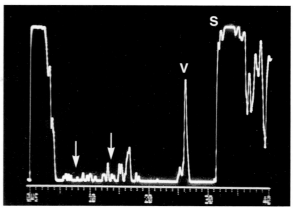

Figure 4.36 Quantitative A-scan of PVD associated with vitreous haemorrhage. The haemorrhage is represented by the low reflective spikes (arrow). The posterior hyaloid face (V) appears as a thin-peaked 60% tall spike (compared to the scleral signal, S)

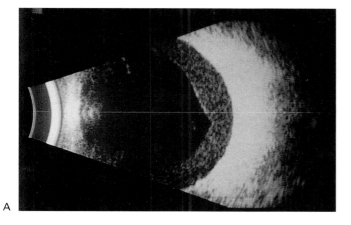

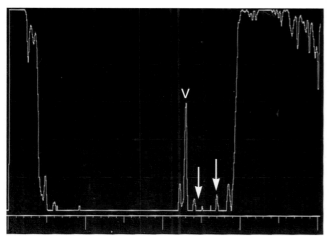

Figure 4.35 Transverse B- and A-scans of a PVD associated with subhyaloid haemorrhage. In the B-scan (Figure 4.35A), the detached posterior vitreous face demarcates a clear intra-gel cavity from a subhyaloid space containing dispersed haemorrhage. This is also seen on A-scan (Figure 4.35B) where, unlike the clear vitreous cavity, the subhyaloid space contains a weak chain of spikes (arrows) representing haemorrhage. The detached posterior hyaloid (V) shows a 50% spike height

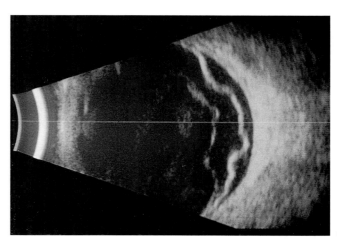

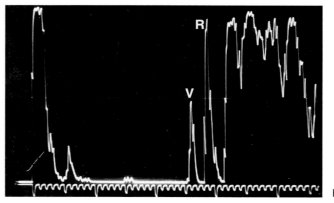

Figure 4.37 Quantitative assessment of PVD and retinal detachment. The B-scan (Figure 4.37A) shows the PVD as a thin linear opacity, in comparison to the more folded and thicker retinal detachment. The two opacities are better quantified on A-scan (Figure 4.37B) with the PVD producing a 50% tall spike (V) compared to the 100% tall retinal spike (R)

can produce a thick, 80–90% tall spike, mimicking retinal detachment. Differentiation can be assisted in these cases by measuring the difference in decibels between the 50% spike height of the membrane in question and that of the sclera – a method described by Ossoinig as 'quantitative echography type II' (Figure 4.38).[7]

On *kinetic* evaluation, PVD is more mobile, during and after termination of eye movement, compared to retinal and choroidal detachment. The vitreous spike on A-scan exhibits excessive lateral and vertical shifts (Figure 4.7). The kinetic examination also includes assessment of the vitreo-retinal relation, particularly at the potential areas of adhesions described above.

The characteristic features of the three membranous opacities are summarized in Table 4.1.

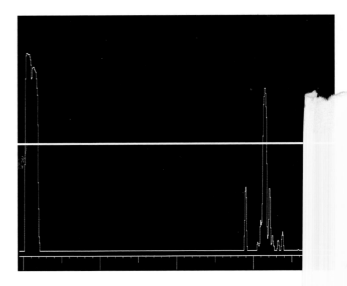

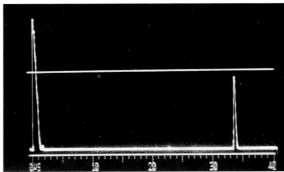

Figure 4.38 'Quantitative echography II.' In Figure 4.38 A, th[e] is reduced to 32 dB. Two spikes are displayed: one (the PVD) b[elow] the 50% reference line and one (sclera) above the line. In Figur[e] the gain is further reduced to 11.5; only the scleral signal is dis[played] up to the 50% reference line. The difference in decibels betwee[n] 50% reflectivity of the sclera and the membrane in question ca[n] the diagnosis (for the retina it is 15 dB or less, for PVD 20 dB o[r]

Table 4.1 Special examination techniques: intraocular membrane			
Examination	Choroidal detachment	Retinal detachment	PVD*
Topographic (B) Shape	Dome-shaped	Linear V	V U
Location	Periphery (pre-equator)	Variable	Variable
Attachment to optic nerve	No	Yes	Variable
Other	Kissing choroids Vortex vein	Folds Breaks	Thicker inferiorly
Quantitaive (A) Spike height	90–100%	80–100%	40–90%
Spike peak	Double	Single	Single
Kinetic (A and B) Mobility	Minimal	Moderate	Marked
After-movement	Absent	Minimal to moderate	Marked
*PVD = posterior vitreous detachment.			

INTRAOCULAR TUMOURS

The differentiation between choroidal melanoma, metastasis, choroidal haemangioma, and other mimicking lesions can be greatly improved if all possible A- and B- scan data are collected. The value of echographic examination is particularly evident in opaque media. But even when fundoscopy is possible, the addition of echographic findings to the clinical and other investigative data is likely to secure a correct diagnosis in a high percentage of cases and deliver the appropriate treatment, particularly if enucleation is contemplated.

Uveal melanoma

In the *topographic* examination, choroidal melanoma appears as a smooth dome (Figure 4.39) or, more characteristically, as a mushroom-shaped solid mass as it

breaks through Bruch's membrane (Figure 4.40). Less frequently, large choroidal melanomas may exhibit an irregular outline (Figure 4.41), and may rarely present as a diffuse, mild thickening of the choroid extending

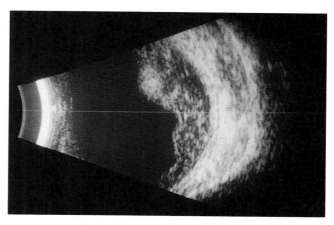

Figure 4.41 A large choroidal melanoma occupying an extensive area of the fundus, showing an irregular, multi-dome surface

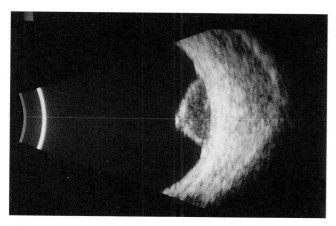

Figure 4.39 B-scan appearance of a dome-shaped choroidal melanoma. A degree of 'choroidal excavation' is also demonstrated

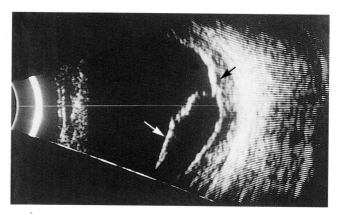

Figure 4.42 A choroidal melanoma, unusually presenting as diffuse thickening of the choroid over a large area (black arrow), and associated with an area of retinal detachment (white arrow)

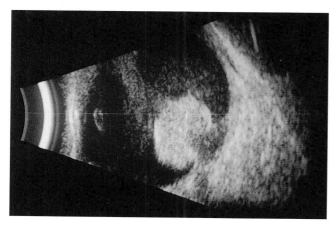

Figure 4.40 Longitudinal B-scan showing the characteristic mushroom or collar-stud appearance of choroidal melanoma. A moderately dense vitreous haemorrhage is also seen, which is likely to have prevented adequate ophthalmoscopy

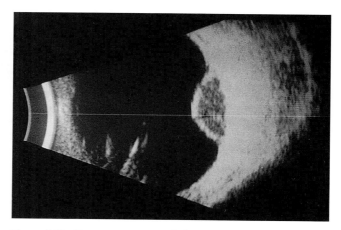

Figure 4.43 B-scan appearance of 'choroidal excavation'. A smooth, dome-shaped melanoma is demonstrated. The line of the globe wall behind the tumour appears to be punched out or excavated, as compared to the globe wall on either side of the tumour

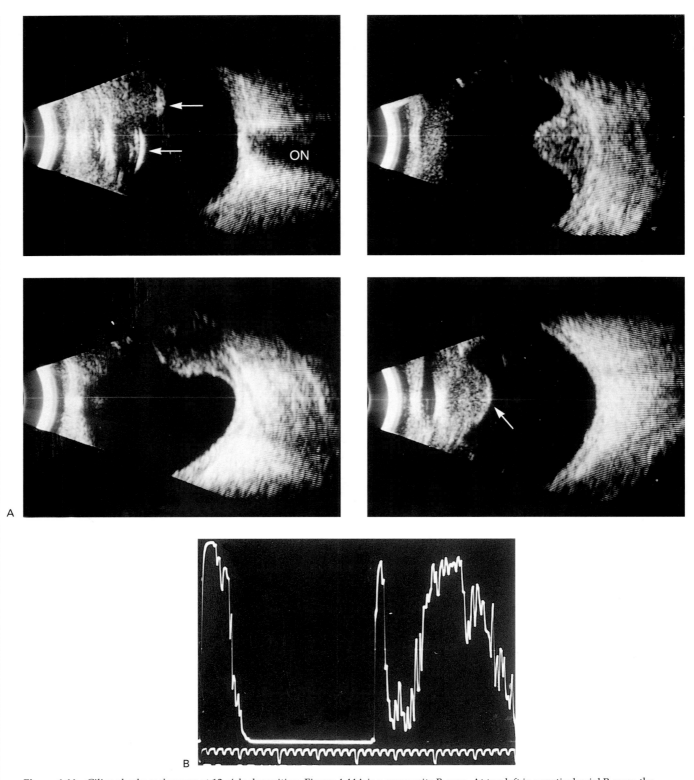

Figure 4.44 Ciliary body melanoma at 12 o'clock position. Figure 4.44A is a composite B-scan. At top left is a vertical axial B-scan: the tumour (top arrow) is seen above the lens (bottom arrow) (ON = optic nerve). At top right is a transverse 12A showing a dome-shaped tumour in the centre of the echogram. At bottom left is a longitudinal scan, and at bottom right a 'direct' scan. In this, the tumour is placed immediately following the initial echoes (arrow). Figure 4.44B is an A-scan; the tumour is predominantly low-reflective but displays a degree of irregularity in its internal structure – a feature commonly seen in ciliary body melanomas

over a wide area (Figure 4.42).[8] A dome-shaped tumour centred in the beam path may produce the well-known 'choroidal excavation' (Figure 4.43).[9] This, however, is not specific to melanoma, but is occasionally seen in other solid, dome-shaped fundus mass lesions.[10] Melanomas can occupy any part of the fundus, including the ciliary body (Figure 4.44), and may be associated with retinal detachment and/or vitreous haemorrhage (Figure 4.40).[11] Careful scanning of the entire tumour base is important to exclude extrascleral extension (Figure 4.45), a significant prognostic finding likely to be missed on clinical examination and fluorescein angiography. Precise localization of the tumour is undertaken on B-scan by the performing of

transverse, longitudinal, and axial sections. The lateral (base) dimensions are obtained from B-scans, and accurate measurement of the tumour height is performed on A-scan at 'measuring sensitivity' (Figure 4.46). Precise documentation and measurement are required for follow-up studies of tumour growth, for monitoring the effect of radiotherapy, and for the accurate placement of radiation plaques.

Quantitative examination involves A-scan assessment of reflectivity, internal structure, and sound attenuation. Malignant melanoma produces low-medium reflective, regularly structured lesion spikes, with medium to high sound attenuation (Figures 4.11, 4.13, 4.46). These features appear to be related to the histo-

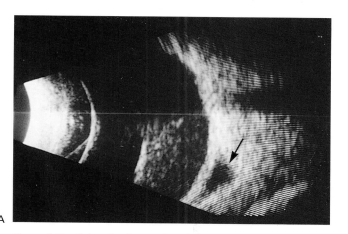
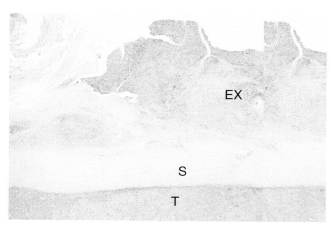

Figure 4.45 Extrascleral extension of choroidal melanoma. The axial B-scan (Figure 4.45A) shows a dome-shaped melanoma occupying the macular area. A low-reflective 'pocket' of extra-scleral extension is seen in the adjacent retrobulbar fat (arrow). Note that the sclera is still 'echographically' intact. These findings were confirmed on histological examination of the enucleated eye (Figure 4.45B). T = tumour, S = sclera, EX = extrascleral extension

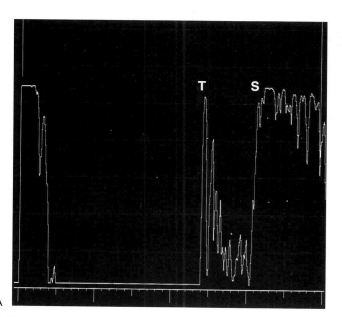
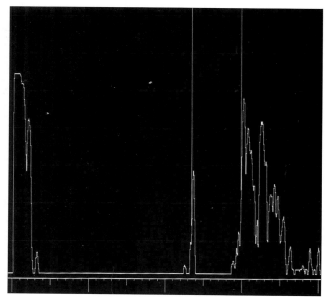

Figure 4.46 A-scan measurement of tumour height. In Figure 4.46A, optimum (perpendicular) trace of the tumour is first obtained at T-sensitivity gain. Note the tall, steeply rising tumour surface spike (T) and scleral spike (S), indicating perpendicularity. In Figure 4.46B, the decibel gain is reduced. The height of the tumour is measured by aligning the electronic callipers (vertical lines) with the peaks of the two spikes

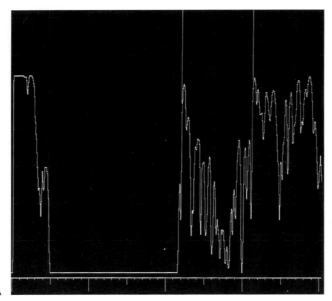
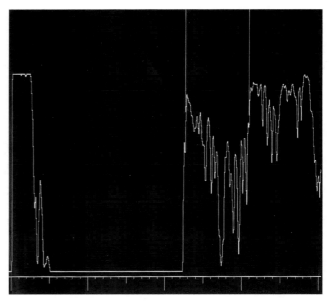

A   B

Figure 4.47 Effect of irradiation on the internal structure of melanomas. Figure 4.47A is the pre-irradiation A-scan of a choroidal melanoma. Figure 4.47B is the appearance 10 months after irradiation. Note the net increase in reflectivity of tumour echoes (between the two vertical lines). Both echograms were taken using the same instrument and decibel (T-sensitivity) gain

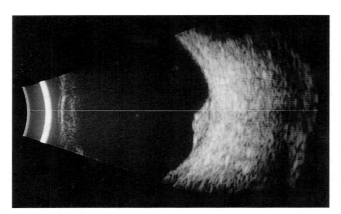
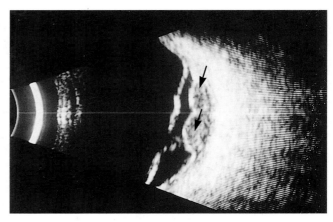

Figure 4.48 B-scan showing a dome-shaped choroidal metastasis with a slightly irregular tumour surface. The B-scan appearance could be mistaken for a melanoma

Figure 4.49 A bi-domed choroidal metastasis from breast carcinoma presenting with retinal detachment (arrows.) The bi-domed configuration is a common feature of metastatic lesions

logical arrangement, i.e. small, tightly packed cells with no large interfaces.[4] The various cell types, however, cannot be differentiated using current techniques and instruments. More irregular internal structure is occasionally encountered in large necrotic choroidal tumours and in melanomas of the ciliary body (Figure 4.44). Radiated tumours also tend to alter their internal structure, with an overall increase in reflectivity (Figure 4.47). This is due to the ensuing necrosis and fibrosis within the tumour.[12,13]

On *kinetic* A-scan, the tumour surface spike shows no movement; this differentiates it from other 'non-solid' lesions. A separate mobile retinal spike may, however, be encountered if the tumour is associated with retinal detachment. In such cases, measurement of tumour height should be taken from the tumour surface and not the retinal spike. Fine, fast, vertical oscillation of some echoes within the tumour mass, indicative of vascularity, is normally seen, and is considered diagnostic of malignant melanoma (Figure 4.9).[2,3,4]

Choroidal metastasis

On *topographic* B-scan evaluation, choroidal metastases can look similar to melanomas (Figure 4.48). Occasionally they exhibit a 'bi-domed' configuration (Figure 4.49), and more commonly an irregular outline (Figure 4.50). Their most common location is in the posterior pole, in the vicinity of the macula, presum-

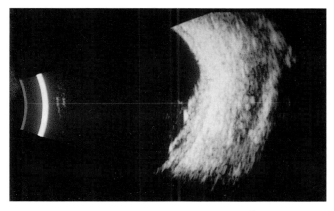

Figure 4.50 A more typical B-scan appearance of choroidal metastasis. The tumour has an irregular outline and an heterogeneous internal structure

ably where malignant cells enter the eye via the short posterior ciliary arteries. Choroidal metastases are rarely associated with vitreous haemorrhage, but tend to cause early and extensive retinal detachment. Bilateral presentation is not uncommon, and follow-up studies usually illustrate rapid growth of the tumour.

Quantitative examination on A-scan shows a variable reflectivity depending on the source of the primary lesion and the arrangement of cell clusters and fibrous septi. The internal structure is therefore irregular, and the sound attenuation is weak (Figure 4.51).

Kinetic examination reveals a solid tumour surface spike. Vascularity in metastasis is normally absent, but has been reported in some cases.[14,15]

Choroidal haemangioma

Topographically choroidal haemangioma may appear as a dome-shaped solid lesion, indistinguishable from

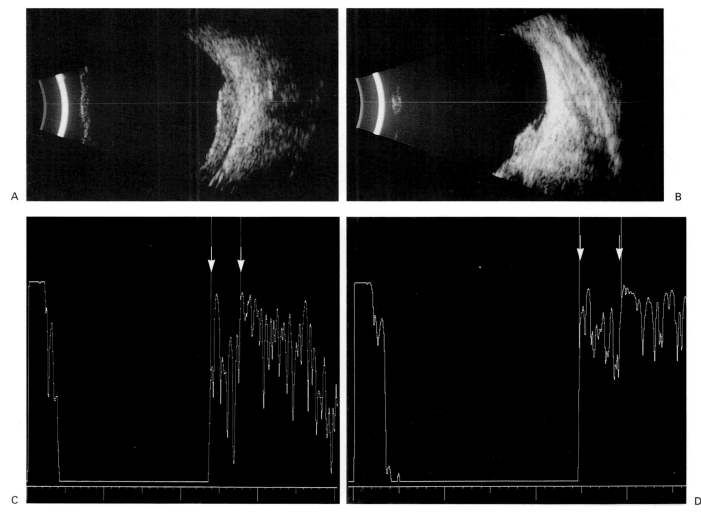

Figure 4.51 B-scans (Figures 4.51A and 4.51B) and A-scans (Figures 4.51C and 4.51D) of two choroidal metastases from two different patients. Note the irregular internal structure and increased reflectivity on A-scans (areas between arrows)

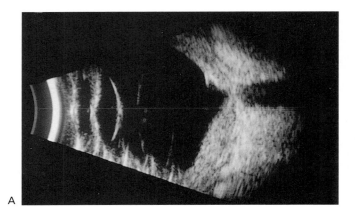

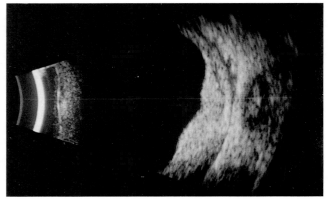

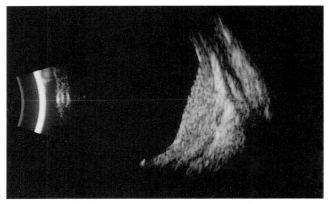

Figure 4.52 Choroidal haemangioma appearing as marked, diffuse, 'granular' choroidal thickening, and occupying a large area of the posterior pole up to the equator. Figure 4.52A shows an axial B-scan, Figure 4.52B a transverse section, and Figure 4.52C a longitudinal section of the lesion

melanoma, or as a marked, diffuse thickening of the retino-choroid layer (Figure 4.52). The most frequent location is in the posterior pole, particularly near the optic disc. Haemangiomas tend to grow very slowly and rarely produce retinal detachment, but localized cystic retinal changes may be seen in long-standing cases.

Quantitaive examination shows a highly reflective, regularly structured tissue, producing weak attenuation (Figure 4.53). This appears to correlate well with the 'honeycomb' histological arrangement of blood-filled loculi separated by thin fibrous septi.

On *kinetic* examination, choroidal haemangiomas are 'echographically' non-vascular, as the large honeycomb spaces are mostly filled with stagnant blood, with no significant blood flow.

The echographic findings for the three tumours are summarized in Table 4.2.

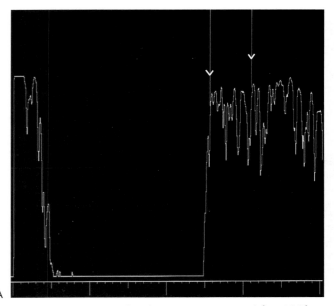

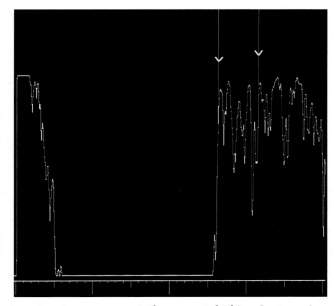

Figure 4.53 Two examples of A-scan appearance of choroidal haemangioma (area between arrows). The tumour is highly reflective and regularly structured and produces weak sound attenuation, i.e. no significant decline in spikes' height from left to right

Table 4.2 Special examination techniques: intraocular tumours

Examination	Melanoma	Metastasis	Haemangioma
Topographic (B)			
Shape	Domed Mushroom	Domed/Bi-domed Irregular	Domed
Location	Variable	Near macula	Near disc
Associated retinal detachment	Variable	Common	Rare
Growth	Variable	Rapid	Slow
Quantitative (A)			
Reflectivity	Low/medium	Variable	High
Internal structure	Regular	Irregular	Regular
Sound attenuation	Strong	Variable	Weak
Kinetic (A)			
Vascularity	Present	Absent	Absent

REFERENCES

1. Guthoff R F, Berger R W, Winkler P et al. Doppler ultrasonography of malignant melanoma of the uvea. Arch Ophthalmol 1991; 109:537–541

2. Hodes B L, Choromokos E. Standardized A-scan echographic diagnosis of choroidal malignant melanoma. Arch Ophthalmol 1977; 95:593–597

3. Ossoinig K C. Advances in diagnostic ultrasound. In: Henkind P (ed) ACTA XXIV International Congress of Ophthalmology. Philadelphia: Lippincott, 1983:89–114

4. Shammas H J. Atlas of ophthalmic ultrasonography and biometry. St Louis: Mosby, 1984:64–70

5. Blumenkranz M S, Byrne S F. Standardized Echography (ultrasonography) for the detection and characterization of retinal detachment. Ophthalmology 1982; 89:821–831

6. Ossoinig K C, Islas G, Tamayo G E et al. Detached retina versus dense fibrovascular membrane: standardized A-scan and B-scan criteria. In: Ossoinig K C (ed) Ophthalmic echography. Dordrecht: Junk, 1987:275

7. Ossoinig K C. Quantitative echography – the basis of tissue differentiation. J of Clin Ultrasound 1974; 2:33–46

8. Font R L, Spaulding A B, Zimmerman L E. Diffuse malignant melanoma of the uveal tract: a clinicopathologic report of 54 cases. Trans Am Acad Ophthalmol Otolaryngol 1968; 72:877–895

9. Coleman D J, Abramson D H, Jack R L et al. Ultrasonic diagnosis of tumours of the choroid. Arch Ophthalmol 1974; 91:344–354

10. Fuller D G, Snyder W B, Hutton W L et al. Ultrasonographic features of choroidal malignant melanoma. Arch Ophthalmol 1979; 97:1465–1472

11. Cunliffe I A, Rennie I G. Choroidal melanoma presenting as vitreous haemorrhage. Eye 1993; 7:711–713

12. Saornil M A, Egan K M, Gragoudas E S et al. Histopathology of proton beam-irradiated vs enucleated uveal melanomas. Arch Ophthalmol 1992; 110:1112–1118

13. Gragoudas E S, Egan K M, Saornil M A et al. The time course of irradiation changes in proton beam-treated uveal melanomas. Ophthalmology 1993; 100:1555–1559

14. Byrne S F, Green R L. Ultrasound of the eye and orbit. St Louis: Mosby Year Book, 1992:175

15. Verbeek A M. A choroidal oat-cell carcinoma metastasis mimicking a choroidal melanoma. In: Thijssen J M, Verbeek A M (eds) Ultrasonography in Ophthalmology. Dordrecht: Junk, 1981:131

5

Biometry of axial eye length and corneal thickness

The ultrasonographic measurement of axial eye length (biometry) and corneal thickness (pachymetry) have become two indispensable ultrasonic investigations following the popularization of intraocular lens implantation and corneal refractive surgery.

The importance of accurate estimation of the dioptric power of the intraocular lens (IOL) is highlighted by the report that Harold Ridley's historical first implant in 1949 produced a postoperative refraction of -18.00^{DS} $-6.00^{C} \times 150°$.[1] The initial resistance to Ridley's pioneering work delayed the wider use of IOLs and the demand for axial eye length measurement. Prior to the introduction of ultrasonic biometry, early implant surgeons relied on data from preoperative refraction to estimate the desired dioptric power of IOL; an example of this is the 'Shepard's Graph' (Figure 5.1).

In 1967, Fyodorov described the first ultrasonic measurement of axial eye length for the purpose of calculating intraocular lens power.[2,3] Using a 'theoretical formula', he incorporated the axial eye length and keratometry reading to estimate the implant power.

Since then a number of theoretical formulae have been added, notably those by Binkhorst,[4] Colenbrander,[5] Thijssen,[6] and Van der Heijde,[7] all based on the schematic eye and including in their calculation the axial eye length, keratometry reading, and estimated postoperative anterior chamber depth. In 1982 a 'regression analysis' method was introduced by Sanders, Retzlaff, and Kraff, commonly known as the 'SRK formula'.[1,8,9] The regression analysis is based on retrospective computer analysis of a large number of

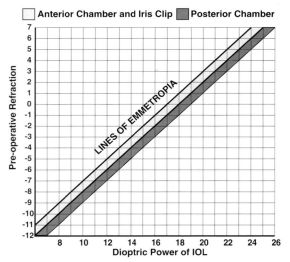

Figure 5.1 Shepard's Graph. One of the 'non-biometric' methods of estimating the dioptre power of intraocular lenses from preoperative refraction. Wider scatter around the line of emmetropia was to be expected

postoperative refractions. Unlike the theoretical formulae, postoperative anterior chamber depth is not included, but is replaced by a constant that is dependent on the type of implant and the technique of the individual surgeon. More recently, further modifications to the SRK formula have been recommended, i.e. the SRK II[10] and SRK/T.[11] A new three-part system, incorporating a theoretical formula, has also been developed by Holladay et al[12] (see Box 5.1), aiming to improve the results in abnormally long and short eyes.

HOLLADAY FORMULAS AND CONSTANTS

Recommended constants

n_c = refractive index of cornea = 4/3
n_a = refractive index of aqueous = 1.336
RT = retinal thickness factor = 0.200 mm

Measured values

K = average K-reading (dioptres)
R = average corneal radius (mm) = 337.5/K
AL = measured ultrasonic axial length (mm)

Chosen values

V = vertex distance of pseudophakic spectacles (mm), default = 12 mm
Ref = desired postoperative spheroequivalent refraction (dioptres)
SF = 'surgeon factor' = distance from aphakic anterior iris plane to optical plane of IOL (mm)

Definitions of other variables

AG = anterior chamber diameter from angle to angle (mm)
ACD = anatomic anterior chamber depth (mm), distance from corneal vertex to anterior iris plane
Alm = modified axial length (mm) = ultrasonic axial length (AL) + retinal thickness factor (RT)
I = power of IOL (dioptres)
ARef = actual postoperative spheroequivalent refraction (dioptres)

EQUATIONS

Eq 1 Rag $= R$, if $R < 7$ mm, then Rag $= 7$ mm
Eq 2 AG $= 12.5 \, AL/23.45$, if $AG > 13.5$ mm, then $AG = 13.5$ mm
Eq 3 ACD $= 0.56 + Rag - (SQRT (Rag \, Rag - (AG \, AG/4)))$

IOL power (I) from desired postoperative refraction (Ref)

Eq 4 $I = \dfrac{1000 \, n_a \, (n_a R - (n_c - 1) \, Alm - 0.001 \, Ref \, (V(n_a R - (n_c - 1) \, Alm) + Alm \, R))}{(Alm - ACD - SF) \, (n_a R - (n_c - 1) \, (ACD + SF) - 0.001 \, Ref \, (V \, (n_a R - (n_c - 1) \, (ACD + SF) + (ACD + SF) \, R))}$

Resultant refraction (Ref) from IOL power (I)

Eq 5 $Ref = \dfrac{1000 \, n_a \, (n_a R - (n_c - 1) \, Alm) - I \, (Alm - ACD - SF) \, (n_a R - (n_c - 1) \, (ACD + SF))}{n_a \, (V \, (n_a R - (n_c - 1) \, Alm) + Alm \, R) - 0.001 \, I \, (Alm - ACD - SF) \, (V \, (n_a R - (n_c - 1) \, (ACD + SF)) + (ACD + SF) \, R)}$

**Reverse solution: 'surgeon factor' (SF) from IOL power (I)
and actual stabilized postoperative refraction (ARef)**

Eq 6 AQ $= (n_c - 1) - (0.001 \, ARef \, ((V \, (n_c - 1)) - R))$
Eq 7 BQ $= ARef \, 0.001 \, ((Alm \, V \, (n_c - 1)) - (R \, (Alm - (V \, n_a)))) - (((n_c - 1) \, Alm) + (n_a R))$
Eq 8 CQ_1 $= 0.001 \, ARef \, ((V \, ((n_a R) - ((n_c - 1) \, Alm))) + (Alm \, R))$
Eq 9 CQ_2 $= (1000 \, n_a \, ((n_a R) - ((n_c - 1) \, Alm) - CQ_1))/I$
Eq 10 CQ_3 $= (Alm \, n_a \, R) - (.001 \, ARef \, Alm \, V \, R \, n_a)$
Eq 11 CQ $= CQ_3 - CQ_2$
Eq 12 SF $= (((-BQ) - SQRT \, ((BQ \, BQ) - (4 \, AQ \, CQ)))/(2 \, AQ)) - ACD$

Numeric example

K	= 46 D	V	= 12 mm	Ref	= − 0.50000 D
AL	= 22 mm	I	= 21.45970 D	ARef	= − 0.50000 D
Alm	= 22.2 mm			SF	= + 0.50000 mm

Forward solution for 'I' and 'Ref'   Reverse solution for 'SF'

Rag	= R = 7.33696 mm	AQ	= .331665	CQ_3 = 218.91391
AG	= 11.72708 mm	BQ	= − 17.22395	CQ = 63.39617
ACD	= 3.48676 mm	CQ_1	= − 0.095853	SF = + 0.50000 mm
I	= 21.45970 D	CQ_2	= 155.51774	
Ref	= − 0.50000 D			

Reproduced with permission from J Cataract Refract Surg 13 January 1988.

Box 5.1

At present the SRK formula (and its modifications) and Holladay's system are probably the most widely used formulae for IOL calculation. More formulae, however, are likely to be added in the future.

As this book is a practical guide to examination methods, more emphasis will be placed on the techniques of axial length measurement and pachymetry. The reader may wish to consult other publications on the merits of the various formulae used to estimate IOL power.[13,14,15] Table 5.1 presents some of the common formulae.

Table 5.1 Examples of formulae for IOL power calculation

Fyodorov's $\quad P = \dfrac{1336 - LK}{(L - C)\,1 - \dfrac{CK}{1336}}$

Colenbrander's $\quad P = \dfrac{1336}{L - C - 0.05} - \dfrac{1336}{\dfrac{1336}{K} - C - 0.05}$

Binkhorst's $\quad P = \dfrac{1336\,(4R - L)}{(L - C)\,(4R - C)}$

SRK's $\quad P = A - 2.5\,L - 0.9\,K$

P = Implant power in diopters.
A = Constant, specific for each type of lens.
C = Estimated postoperative anterior chamber depth (mm).
L = Axial eye length (mm).
K = Avarage keratometry (dioptres).
R = Corneal radius of curvature (mm).

TECHNIQUES OF AXIAL LENGTH MEASUREMENT

The globe lends itself well to accurate ultrasonic measurement. The velocity of sound in the eye and its individual structures is now well known (Table 5.2).[16,17,18]

The cornea, lens, and retina produce good landmarks for perpendicular and axial alignment of the A-scan beam (Figure 5.2) – an essential prerequisite for accurate measurement of the axial eye length. It is recognized that a 1 mm error of axial length measurement results in a 3 dioptre error in postoperative refraction.

In contrast to diagnostic A-scan, biometry scanners do not need to be 'standardized'. A frequency of 10 MHz is commonly employed and the sound beam may be focused or parallel (Figure 5.3). All modern instruments contain automatic freeze frame facilities with an additional option of semi-automatic and manual modes. The latter may be the method of choice in abnormally long and short eyes and measurements in aphakia and pseudophakia.

Biometry and keratometry should ideally be performed by a trained operator who is familiar with the instruments. Examination should be conducted in a quiet room, preferably one solely designated for such purposes. The A-scan and keratometry instruments are best located nearby, allowing a fast and comfortable procedure. It is also helpful if B- and standardized A-scan instruments are easily accessible in case an abnormal signal is detected on biometry A-scan, or a good trace is difficult to obtain.

Two techniques are available for axial length measurement, immersion technique and contact technique.

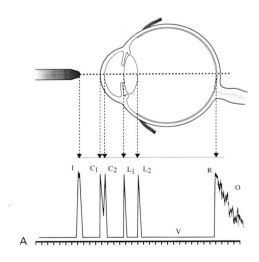

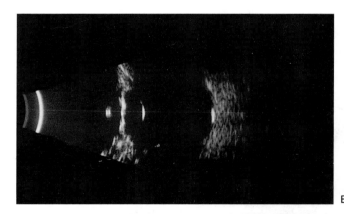

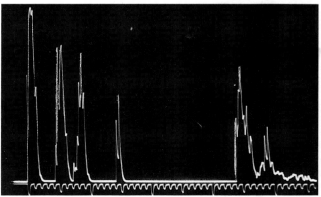

Figure 5.2 Immersion axial scanning of the eye. Figure 5.2A shows how axial alignment of the sound beam can easily be obtained and verified by the observation of equally tall and smooth signals from the anterior corneal surface (C1), posterior corneal surface (C2), anterior lens surface (L1), posterior lens surface (L2), and retina (R). An axial B- and A-scan echogram are shown in Figures 5.2B and 5.2C

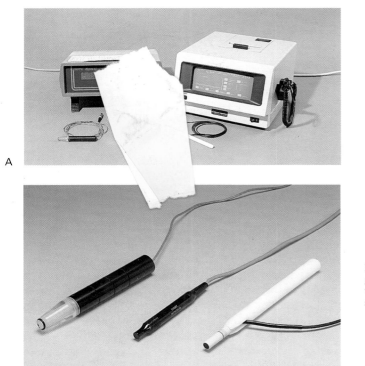

A

B

Figure 5.3 Figure 5.3A: two examples of biometry A-scanners produced by Storz (left) and Allergan Humphry. Figure 5.3B: various probe designs. The probe with water- filled tips (left) is now being replaced with solid tip probes (centre and right) that are easier to maintain

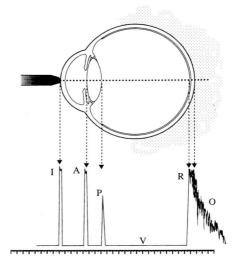

Figure 5.4 Contact A-scan method. The probe is brought into gentle contact with the cornea. The initial spike (I) is now merged with the corneal spikes. A = anterior lens surface, P = posterior lens surface, V = vitreous line, R = retinal spike

Immersion technique

This is arguably the most accurate method, as it eliminates indentation of the cornea. It is, however, more time-consuming, as the patient is required to recline and a water bath needs to be applied. The eye is anaesthetized and a cylindrical hollow shell is inserted under the lids and filled with saline or echo-gel, as described in Chapter 3 (Figures 3.42, 3.43, 3.44). The solution should not be agitated but introduced gently along the shell wall to prevent artefacts from trapped air bubbles. The patient directs the gaze at the primary position, and the probe is inserted into the fluid bath, avoiding corneal contact, and manoeuvred using a high-decibel gain until tall smooth spikes are produced from the cornea, anterior and posterior lens surfaces, and retina (Figure 5.2). The decibel gain is then reduced to approximately 50–60% level, while maintaining perpendicularity, before measurements are taken. Three or more measurements are recorded and averaged.

Contact technique

The probe is placed directly on the anaesthetized cornea with the tear film acting as a sound-transmit-ting medium (Figure 5.4). The least possible pressure should be applied in this technique to prevent undue corneal indentation. Two approaches are possible: applanation and free-standing.

In the applanation method the probe is mounted on an applanation device, on the slit lamp, and the probe is brought into contact with the cornea by the use of the joystick, with application of minimum pressure. Primary gaze orientation may be better achieved in some patients by occluding the fellow eye.

The free-standing method is employed in patients who cannot be positioned on the slit lamp. Care must be taken to prevent undue corneal indentation. The instrument display screen is placed near the patient's head for ease of examination. A distant fixation light may also be helpful in orienting the patient's gaze in the primary position.

In the contact method, the corneal spike is merged with the initial spike, and is therefore replaced by the lens spikes for perpendicular alignment of the sound beam (Figure 5.5). Measurements are taken in a similar way to that used in the immersion technique, i.e. using a medium gain and an average of three or more perpendicular traces. It is important to reduce the decibel gain in order to obtain a more accurate measurement (Figures 5.5, 5.6), and help detect and discard oblique traces.

Biometry in aphakic and pseudophakic eyes

Many biometry instruments contain a function allowing the alteration of sound velocity in certain circumstances (Table 5.2). In the phakic eye a standard sound velocity of 1550 m/s is used. A slight increase in velocity

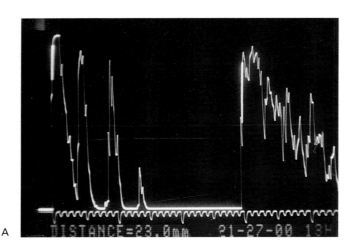

A

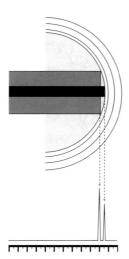

B

Figure 5.5 Contact A-scan. Figure 5.5A: a high-sensitivity axial scan showing the usual landmarks and an axial eye length of 23.00 mm. Figure 5.5B: the same trace after reducing gain by 50%; a more accurate axial measurement is obtained (23.3 mm) (see Figure 5.6)

Table 5.2 Sound velocity in ocular tissues/media	
Tissue	Velocity (m/s)
Globe (phakic)	1550
Globe (aphakic)	1532
Aqueous/vitreous	1532
Cornea	1620
Crystalline lens	1641
Cataractous lens	1629
Sclera	1630
Fat	1476
Silicone oil	986
PMMA	2718

of between 50 and 100 m/s is available in some instruments for dense cataracts.

In the aphakic eye the sound travels at a slower speed, with most instruments employing a figure of 1532 m/s. The two lens spikes are absent in aphakic cases or may be replaced by a single spike of variable height, obtained from the anterior vitreous face and/or posterior lens capsule. Therefore, the immersion technique is the method of choice in aphakic eyes, as it deploys the corneal spike, in place of the lens spikes, to verify perpendicularity and axial alignment (Figure 5.7).

In pseudophakic eyes the calculated sound velocity depends on the implant material. The velocity in PMMA is 2718 m/s. Silicone, however, has a much slower sound velocity, estimated at 986 m/s, giving an average sound velocity of 1486 m/s in pseudophakic eyes implanted with silicone IOLs.[19] The effect of silicone is vividly illustrated on B-scan echograms of eyes filled with silicone oil following vitrectomy, as the eye

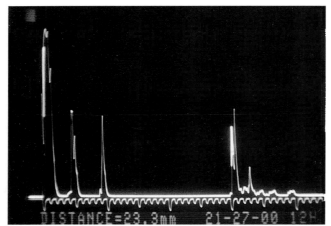

Figure 5.6 The effect of reducing gain on the accuracy of axial length measurement. A high-gain scan produces a wide beam (grey) and an apparently shorter axial length. As the gain is reduced the beam narrows (black), resulting in a more accurate (longer) measurement. Oblique scans will also be easily detected as they produce weak spikes

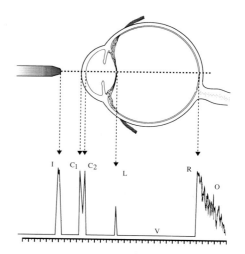

Figure 5.7 Axial length measurement in aphakic eyes. An immersion technique is best utilized as it produces clear corneal spikes (C1 and C2) that help perpendicular alignment. A signal from the posterior capsule (L) is invariably seen. I = initial spike, V = vitreous, R = retina, O = orbital spikes

appears markedly elongated (Figure 5.8). In a recent publication,[20] Holladay and Prager recommended adding 0.4 mm for PMMA and subtracting 0.8 mm for silicone lenses, after estimating the axial eye length using the aphakic velocity (1532 m/s).

Multiple reverberation signals are also encountered in pseudophakic eyes. They are created as the sound waves ricochet back and forth between the probe tip and the highly reflective implant surfaces. In these circumstances the usual landmarks may be difficult to recognize, and reducing the gain will help one better to identify the (relatively high) retinal spike (Figure 5.9).

Practical hints

- Conduct the examination in a quiet, dimly lit room

separate from those used for examining mainstay patients in the clinic or the ward.
- Make sure you understand how the A-scan equipment works, particularly the need to alter sound velocity in aphakic, pseudophakic, and silicone-oil-filled eyes, as well as the position of the measuring gates and gain control.
- In deciding which A-scan to buy, preference should be given to instruments providing good display screens, manual (in addition to automatic) option of trace selection, visible and easy-to-manoeuvre measuring gates, and solid tip probes (Figure 5.3). Most modern instruments will include computing facilities for IOL power calculation. Choose those which are easy to update as more formulae are introduced.
- Conduct keratometry first, before installing local

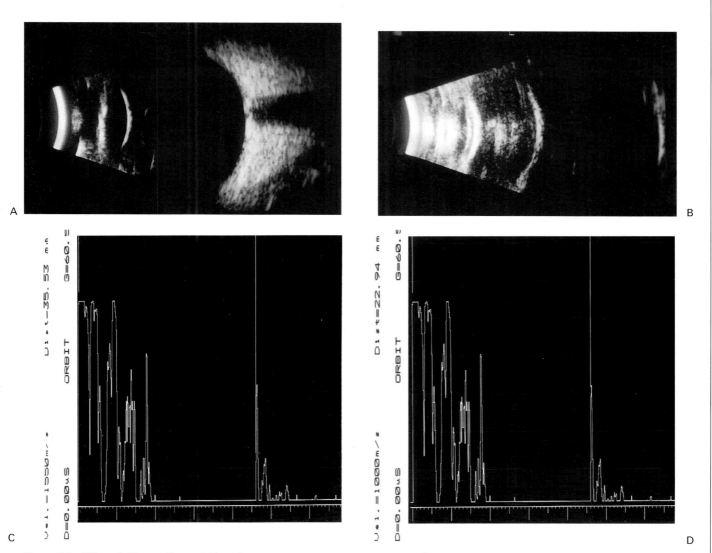

Figure 5.8 Effect of silicone oil on axial length measurement. Figure 58A: B-scan of the fellow normal eye. Figure 5.8B: silicone-filled eye. Note the apparent, marked increase in eye length resulting in loss of orbital image. Figure 5.8C: A-scan using a 'standard' sound velocity of 1550 m/s, giving an erroneous axial length of 35.53 mm. Figure 5.8D: the correct axial length of 22.94 mm is recorded after sound velocity has been reduced to that approximating silicone oil (1000 m/s)

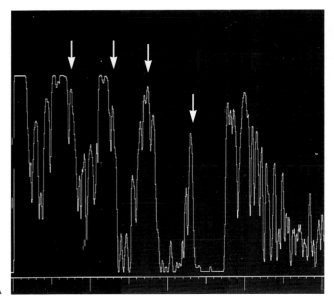

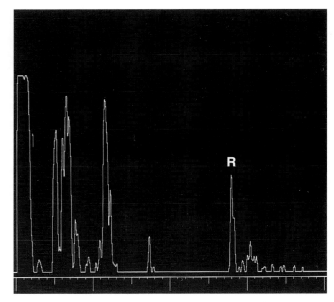

Figure 5.9 Biometry in pseudophakic eyes. Figure 5.9A: high-gain scan showing multiple reverberation signals produced by the IOL (arrows). Figure 5.9B: gain is reduced allowing better identification of the retinal spike (R)

anaesthetic. Ensure that the keratometry instrument is regularly calibrated according to the manufacturer's instructions. A 1 dioptre error in the keratometry reading will result in a 1 dioptre error in postoperative refraction.

- Measure the axial length in both eyes. Symmetrical readings are likely to indicate accurate measurements. Asymmetry of 0.5 mm or more

should be further investigated by repeated measurements and, if necessary, B-scan examination to exclude lesions such as a raised mass or posterior staphyloma. Abnormal vitreous echoes or a weak retinal signal are additional indications for diagnostic A- and B-scan examination (Figure 5.10).

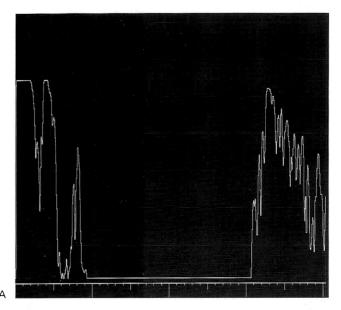

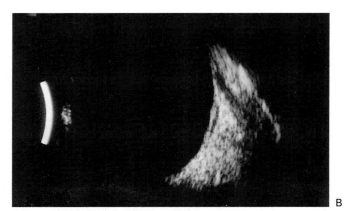

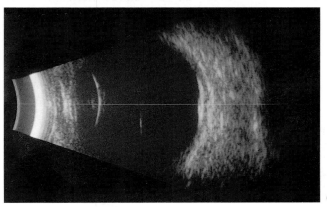

Figure 5.10 Figure 5.10A: an irregular, serrated retinal spike detected during biometry. Figure 5.10B: Macular thickening was found on longitudinal B-scan (arrow). Figure 5.10C: vertical macula scan showing flattening and irregularity at the macular region (arrow)

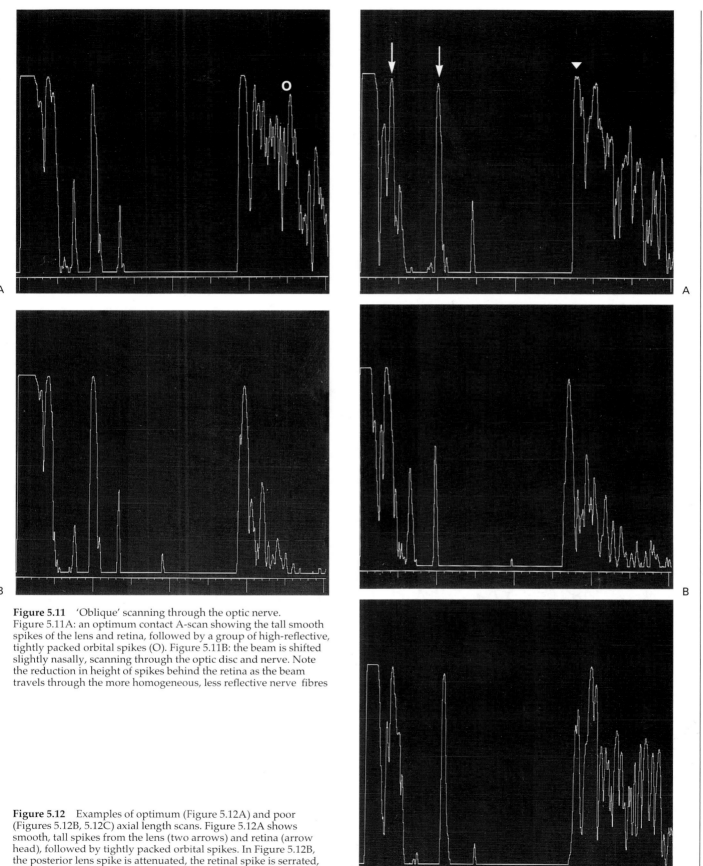

Figure 5.11 'Oblique' scanning through the optic nerve. Figure 5.11A: an optimum contact A-scan showing the tall smooth spikes of the lens and retina, followed by a group of high-reflective, tightly packed orbital spikes (O). Figure 5.11B: the beam is shifted slightly nasally, scanning through the optic disc and nerve. Note the reduction in height of spikes behind the retina as the beam travels through the more homogeneous, less reflective nerve fibres

Figure 5.12 Examples of optimum (Figure 5.12A) and poor (Figures 5.12B, 5.12C) axial length scans. Figure 5.12A shows smooth, tall spikes from the lens (two arrows) and retina (arrow head), followed by tightly packed orbital spikes. In Figure 5.12B, the posterior lens spike is attenuated, the retinal spike is serrated, and the orbital spikes are weak. In Figure 5.12C, the lens spikes are tall but the retinal spike is weak and poorly defined

- Repeat carefully the measurements in abnormally short (less than 22.00 mm) and long (more than 25.00 mm) eyes.
- Beware of 'hitting' the optic disc; a deep cup will produce an erroneously long eye and an elevated disc a short one (Figure 5.11).
- Measurement of the axial eye length with B-scan may be a 'second-best' option in some difficult cases, e.g. patients unable to maintain a steady primary gaze or eyes containing calcified cataract and posterior staphyloma.

Figure 5.12 illustrates three examples of 'good' and 'bad' traces.

OTHER INDICATIONS FOR AXIAL EYE-LENGTH MEASUREMENT

Measurement of the axial eye length is occasionally required in other circumstances, such as in congenital glaucoma, to help reach a diagnosis and monitor the efficacy of treatment.[21] Biometry is useful in eliminating axial myopia and posterior staphyloma as a cause of pseudo-exophthalmos (Figure 5.13), and assists in the diagnosis of microphthalmia and nanophthalmia. The former produces a normal axial eye length with small corneal diameters, and the latter a short axial length and a markedly thickened chorio-retinal layer.

TECHNIQUE OF CORNEAL PACHYMETRY

Measurement of corneal thickness is required in refractive surgery and as an indicator of endothelial cell function.

Pachymetry instruments employ a corneal sound velocity of 1620 m/s. A perpendicular corneal measurement produces two equally tall spikes. Most instruments, however, do not display the echogram but rely on 'computer pattern recognition', in which only spikes with certain height are captured and measured.

The sound velocity is first verified, and a medium-gain setting is used, as high gains may produce unwanted reverberation signals. The eye is anaesthetized and fixation is maintained at the primary position. A central corneal point is first obtained, as this is the key measurement. The test is repeated numerous times. The smallest consistent reading is

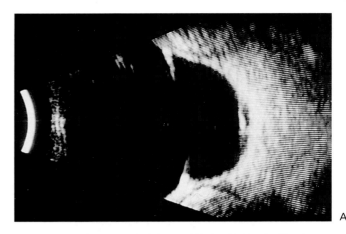

A

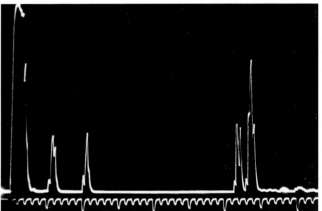

B

Figure 5.13 Posterior staphyloma. Figure 5.13A: B-scan showing a marked posterior pouching of the globe wall in an eye presenting with pseudo-exophthalmos. Figure 5.13B: the axial eye length on A-scan measures 33.9 mm

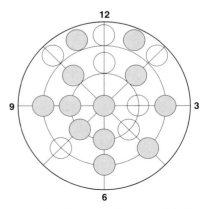

Figure 5.14 Corneal pachymetry. The corneal thickness is first measured at a central point and further points are measured radially or concentrically, depending on the clinical requirement

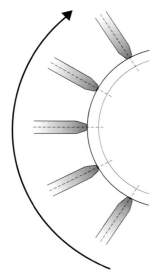

Figure 5.15 Corneal pachymetry. Perpendicularity is maintained by tilting the probe along the corneal curvature

considered the most perpendicular and accurate one. A figure of 500 μm is an average median in most cases.

Depending on the clinical requirement, one central measurement or multiple measurements (corneal mapping) are obtained. This is performed in a radial or concentric fashion around the central point (Figure 5.14). In peripheral measurements the probe is tilted along corneal radii to maintain perpendicularity (Figure 5.15).

As in axial eye-length biometry, pachymetry of the two eyes is important as, in normal circumstance, symmetrical readings would indicate correct measurements.

REFERENCES

1. Retzlaff J, Sanders D, Kraff M. A manual of implant power calculation: SRK Formula. Oregon: Medford 1982:7
2. Fyodorov S N, Kolinko A I. Estimation of optical power of the intraocular lens. Vestik Oftalmol (Moscow) 1967; 4:27–31
3. Fyodorov S N, Galin M A, Linksz A. Calculation of the optical power of intraocular lenses. Invest Ophthalmol 1975; 14:625–628 1975
4. Binkhorst R D. The optical design of intraocular lens implants. Ophthalmic Surg. 1975; 6:17–31
5. Colenbrander M C. Calculation of the power of an iris clip lens for distance vision. Br J Ophthalmol 1973; 57:735–740
6. Thijssen J M. The emmetropic and the iseikonic implant lens: computer calculation of the refractive power and its accuracy. Ophthalmologica 1975; 171:467–486
7. Van der Heijde G L. A nomogram for calculating the power of the prepupillary lens in the aphakic eye. Bibl Ophthalmol 1975; 83:273–275
8. Retzlaff J. A new intraocular lens calculation formula. Am Intra-Ocular Implant Soc J 1980; 6:148–152 1980
9. Sanders D, Kraff M. Improvement of intraocular lens power calculation using empirical data. Am Intra-Ocular Implant Soc J 1980; 6:263–267
10. Sanders D R, Retzlaff J, Kraff M C. Comparison of the SRK II formula and other second generation formulas. J Cataract Refract Surg 1988; 14:136–141
11. Retzlaff J, Sanders D R, Kraff M C. Development of the SRK/T intraocular lens implant power calculation formula. J Cataract Refract Surg 1990; 16:27–33
12. Holladay J T, Prager T C, Chandler T Y et al. A three-part system for refining intraocular lens power calculations. J Cataract Refract Surg 1988; 14:17–24
13. Richards S C, Steen D W. Clinical evaluation of the Holladay and SRK II formulas. J Cataract Refract Surg 1990; 16:71–74
14. Richards S C, Olson R J, Richards W L et al. Clinical evaluation of six intraocular lens calculation formulas. Am Intra-Ocular Implant Soc J 1985; 11:153–158
15. Fritz K J. Intraocular lens power formulas. Am J Ophthalmol 1981; 91:414–415
16. Coleman D J, Lizzi F L, Franzen L A et al. A determination of the velocity of ultrasound in cataractous lenses. In: Gitter K A, Keeney A H, Sarin L K, Meyer D (eds) Ophthalmic ultrasound. St Louis: Mosby, 1969:246
17. Jansson F, Kock E. Determination of the velocity of ultrasound in the human lens and vitreous. Acta Ophthalmologica 1962; 40:420–433
18. Jansson F, Sundmark E. Determination of the velocity of ultrasound in ocular tissues at different temperatures. Acta Ophthalmologica 1961; 39:899
19. Holladay J, Prager T. Accurate ultrasonic biometry in pseudophakia. Am J Ophthalmol 1989; 107:189–190
20. Holladay J, Prager T. Accurate ultrasonic biometry in pseudophakia. Am J Ophthalmol 1993; 115:536–537 1993
21. Massin M, Pellat B. Ultrasonic biometry in congenital glaucoma–a clinical study. In: Hillman J S, Lemay M M (eds) Ophthalmic ultrasound. Dordrecht: Junk, 1984:191

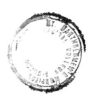

6

Indications: globe

In this section, a summary of the ocular indications for echography will be presented from the clinical standpoint, and the echographic findings for each clinical condition are illustrated. Biometry of the axial eye length and corneal pachymetry are described in Chapter 5. The therapeutic usage of ultrasound is not discussed as it is beyond the remit of this book.

It is to be emphasized that the indications and findings presented are by no mean complete, but serve to illustrate the common applications and diagnoses likely to be encountered. Some of the main echographic features have already been discussed in Chapter 4.

The indications for diagnostic ultrasound in the eye fall into three major categories: opaque media, clear media, ocular trauma.

OPAQUE MEDIA

Dense cataract

Echography is required when fundoscopy is ham-

pered and further abnormalities are suspected, particularly in the presence of additional clinical features such as marked and rapid reduction of vision, a history of trauma, long-standing dense cataract, high myopia, afferent pupillary defect, iris heterochromia and rubeosis, posterior synechia, and diabetes.

Echographic examination of the eye may demonstrate an obvious posterior segment lesion, such as retinal detachment or intraocular tumour. Other 'unexpected' findings include posterior staphyloma (Figure 5.13), optic disc cupping (Figure 6.1), macular thickening (Figure 6.2), and asteroid hyalosis (Figure 6.3). Thickened, intumescent cataracts are easily detected on peripheral B-scan sections (Figure 6.4).

The echographer is able to advise the clinician on the presence of extreme or asymmetrical axial eye lengths or calcification in the cataract which may affect the biometric calculation of intraocular lenses.

Vitreous haemorrhage

The main indication for echography in vitreous haemorrhage is to exclude an underlying retinal tear (Figure 6.5) and retinal detachment (Figures 6.6, 6.7,

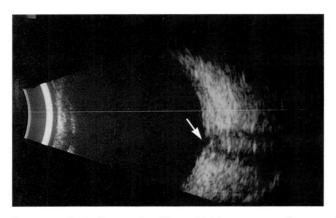
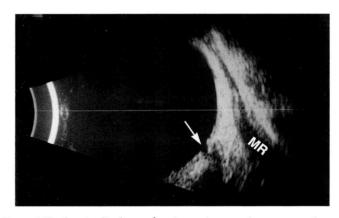

Figure 6.1 Optic disc cupping. Figure 6.1A is a transverse B-scan and Figure 6.1B a longitudinal scan showing an interruption or excavation of the globe wall (arrows) at the optic nerve head. Such an obvious defect would indicate a large (pathological) cup. MR = medial rectus muscle

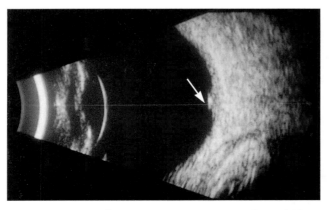
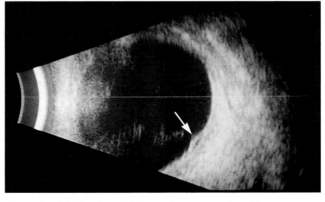

Figure 6.2 Macular thickening. Figure 6.2A: 'vertical macula' B-scan showing a focal thickening at the macular area produced by cystoid macular oedema. Figure 6.2B: longitudinal scan showing a pointed elevation of the macula (arrow) in a case of 'stage III' macular hole

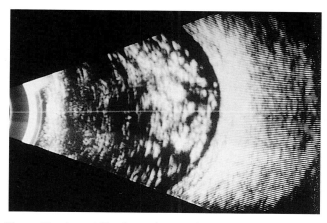
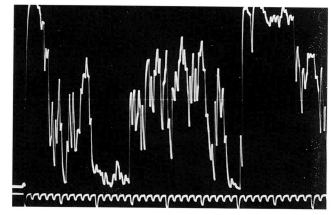

Figure 6.3 Asteroid hyalosis. These are highly reflective opacities, producing characteristic multiple concentric artefacts on B-scan and high-amplitude mobile signals on A-scan. A clear vitreous zone next to the globe wall is usually seen, indicating posterior vitreous detachment

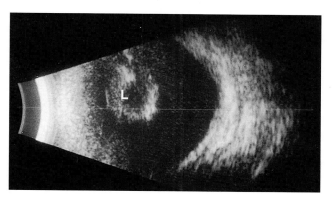
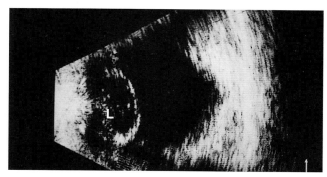

Figure 6.4 Two examples of peripheral, contact B-scans showing thick cataractous lens L. Normal lenses are not so readily seen on such sections

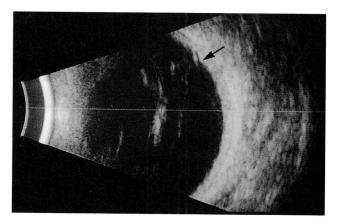
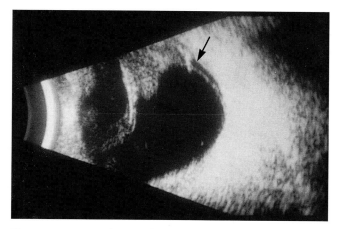

Figure 6.5 Haemorrhagic posterior vitreous detachment (PVD) and retinal tear. Intra-gel echoes (haemorrhage) are seen. The faint line of the detached posterior hyaloid can be traced to an area of vitreo-retinal adhesion where a retinal tear (operculum) is demonstrated (arrow)

Figure 6.6 Vitreous haemorrhage and early retinal detachment. A dense vitreous haemorrhage and high PVD are seen, associated with localized shallow retinal detachment at the temporal periphery (arrow)

6.8). As tears are more frequent in the periphery and superiorly, careful screening of the upper fundus periphery should be performed. Kinetic examination of the vitreous body may show a focal adhesion to the retina, an area of possible retinal tear. The ability to

detect retinal tears depends on the dimensions of the detached retinal leaf and the degree of surrounding subretinal fluid (Figures 6.9, 6.10, 6.11). High-resolution 'eye-dedicated' scanners are likely to be more successful in detecting small tears and shallow peripheral

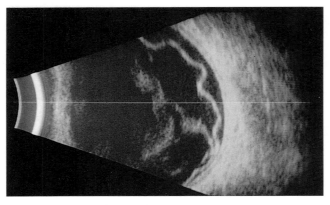

Figure 6.7 Vitreous haemorrhage and extensive retinal detachment. A moderate degree of vitreous haemorrhage is seen. The retina, appearing as a folded line, is extensively detached over a wide area

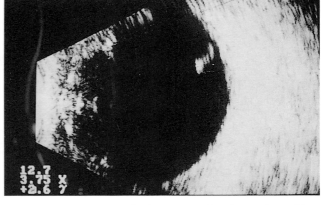

Figure 6.9 Retinal tear with a large operculum but no detectable subretinal fluid

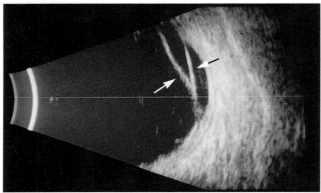

A

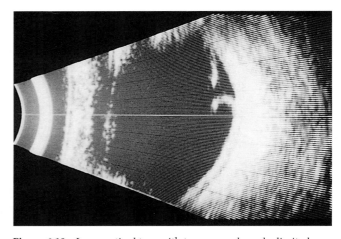

Figure 6.10 Large retinal tear with two opercula and a limited amount of subretinal fluid

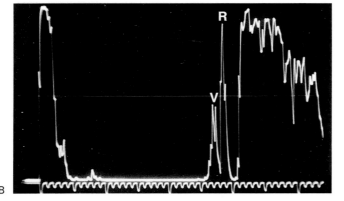

B

Figure 6.8 Vitreous haemorrhage and retinal detachment. The B-scan (Figure 6.8A) shows a mild vitreous haemorrhage, partial PVD (left arrow), and poorly mobile retinal detachment (right arrow). The A-scan (Figure 6.8B) illustrates the vitreo-retinal relation and the difference in reflectivity. V = vitreous spike, R = retinal spike

detached posterior vitreous face, particularly inferiorly (Figure 6.8), as described in Chapter 4.

Another disease frequently associated with vitreous haemorrhage is a bleeding disciform macular lesion (Figure 6.12), which can be paramacular or 'eccentric' disciform – a diagnosis that may not be readily recognized clinically. In such cases A-scan assessment of the reflectivity and internal structure of the lesion is helpful in excluding melanoma.[1] Serial examinations will also show, unlike in cases of metastases, a reduction in the diameter of the lesion.

Other causes of vitreous haemorrhage include bleeding from choroidal melanoma (Figure 6.13),[2] long-standing central retinal vein occlusion, and proliferative diabetic retinopathy.

In diabetic vitreous haemorrhage, single or multiple focal adhesions are frequently seen between incompletely detached posterior vitreous face and 'fibro-vascular' complexes which originate from the optic disc and major retinal vessels. In addition, tractional retinal

retinal detachments. Echo-resolution is further increased by the avoidance of scanning through the lens and by the use of low (decibel) gain settings. Quantitative echography is sometimes required to differentiate between retinal detachment and thick,

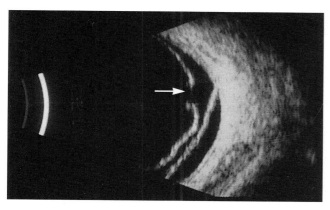
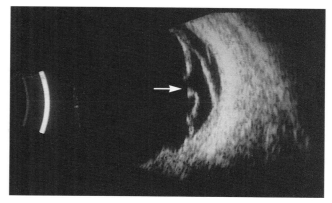

Figure 6.11 Extensive retinal detachment and retinal tear associated with choroidal detachment. Two B-scans taken at right angles to each other show a retinal detachment with a large retinal break (arrow). The choroid is also detached with a clear supra-choroidal space

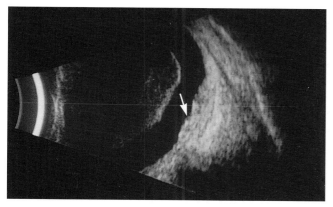

A

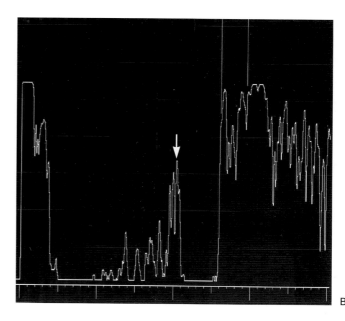

B

Figure 6.12 Bleeding disciform. Figure 6.12A: a longitudinal B-scan showing vitreous haemorrhage, total PVD, and an irregular macular mass (arrow). Figure 6.12B: an A-scan showing a series of low vitreous spikes, limited posteriorly by the PVD spike (arrow). A highly reflective, irregularly structured macular thickening is also demonstrated

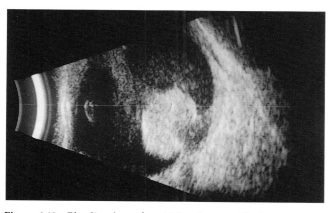

A

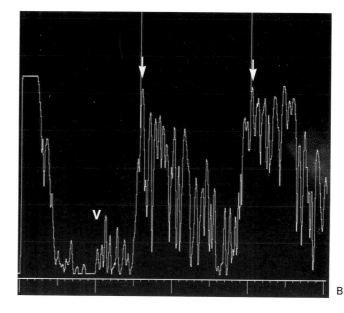

B

Figure 6.13 Bleeding from choroidal melanoma. The B-scan (Figure 6.13A) shows a typical mushroom-shaped melanoma associated with a moderate degree of dispersed vitreous haemorrhage. The A-scan (Figure 6.13B) shows low-amplitude vitreous echoes (V), followed by a large melanoma, measuring 11.22 mm in height (between two arrows)

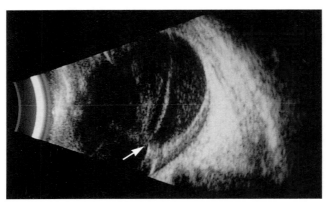

Figure 6.14 Diabetic vitreous haemorrhage: an echogram showing a moderate degree of vitreous haemorrhage and incomplete PVD with a focal vitreo-retinal adhesion (arrow), producing tractional retinal detachment in the macular area

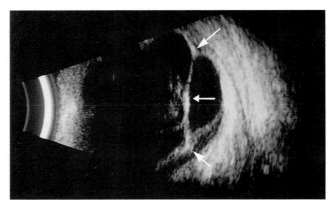

Figure 6.16 Extensive vitreo-retinal adhesions in a diabetic eye. Two foci of tractional retinal detachments are seen (top and bottom arrows). They are bridged by a thick, incompletely detached posterior hyaloid (middle arrow)

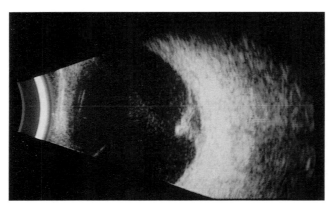

Figure 6.15 Fine diabetic vitreous haemorrhage and a focal tinted retinal detachment produced by firm vitreo-retinal adhesions

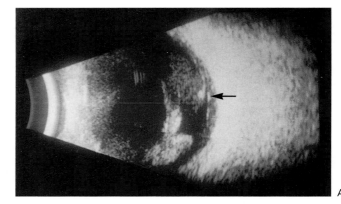

Figure 6.17 B- and A-scans of intra-gel haemorrhage. A large coalescent opacity (clot) is seen on B-scan (Figure 6.17A), which also depicts a shallow, incomplete PVD (arrow). On A-scan (Figure 6.17B) the clot appears as a thick, highly reflective ragged spike (arrow)

detachment(s) may also be found (Figures 6.14, 6.15, 6.16).

Vitreous haemorrhage may be 'spontaneous', with no known associated clinical disease or echographic evidence of a pre-existing lesion.[3,4] Repeat ultrasound examinations are indicated in such cases to detect early retinal detachment and other abnormalities.[5]

Haemorrhage into the vitreous tends to form clots. These appear as highly reflective, coalescent echoes (Figure 6.17), which are usually denser inferiorly. Bleeding associated with posterior vitreous detachment may be confined to the gel (Figure 6.18) or sub-hyaloid space alone (Figure 6.19), or may be mixed (Figure 6.20). Subhyaloid haemorrhage associated with posterior vitreous detachment should raise the suspicion of a retinal tear, especially in an otherwise healthy eye or in high myopia.

Unlike intra-gel haemorrhage, subhyaloid haemorrhage does not clot, and appears therefore as dispersed, mobile small echoes, requiring a high gain setting to be demonstrated. Chronic, subhyaloid

haemorrhage may gravitate inferiorly, forming an interface between a thick, highly reflective layer of blood and less dense floating blood cells (Figures 6.21, 6.22). This thick layer, commonly known as 'posterior

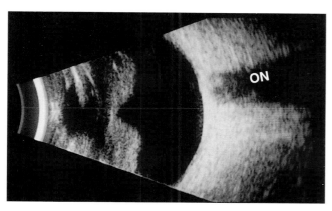
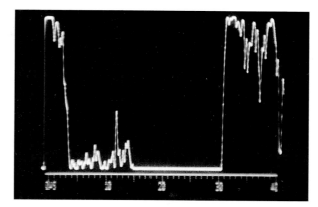

Figure 6.18 B- and A-scans of dense vitreous haemorrhage and high, complete PVD. The haemorrhage is confined to the vitreous with a clear, echo-silent retro-hyaloid space. ON = optic nerve

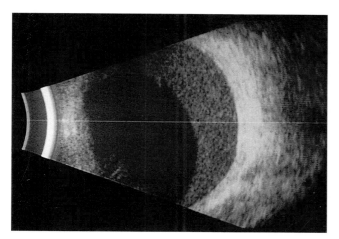

Figure 6.19 B-scan showing clear vitreous space and PVD. The subhyaloid space is completely filled with fine, dispersed opacities representing fluid blood

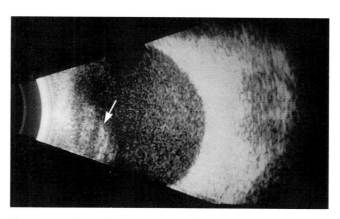

Figure 6.20 A mixed intra-gel and subhyaloid haemorrhage in an aphakic eye. The arrow points to a high PVD and posterior vitreous face

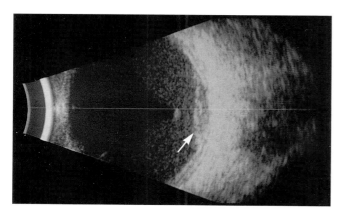

Figure 6.21 Posterior hyphaema. The scan shows a faint subhyaloid haemorrhage and a well-outlined, dense opacity overlaying the globe wall (arrow), representing a thicker layer of blood

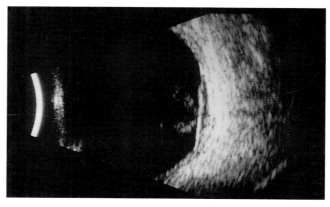

Figure 6.22 Another example of posterior hyphaema. On kinetic echography the fluid level can be made to slide along the globe wall, confirming the diagnosis and ruling out solid mass lesion

hyphaema',[6,7] can be made to slide along the globe wall with eye movements; this distinguishes it from mimicking (solid) thickening of the retino-choroid layer.

Leukokoria

The safety and ease of access of ultrasound, and the fact that it can be performed during examination under anaesthetic (EUA), make it an ideal tool in the investigation of children with leukokoria.[8,9,10,11] In most of these cases, fundoscopy is difficult to perform owing to media opacities, poor pupillary dilatation, and lack of patient cooperation.

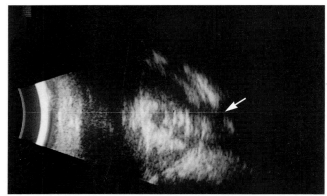

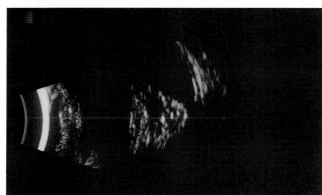

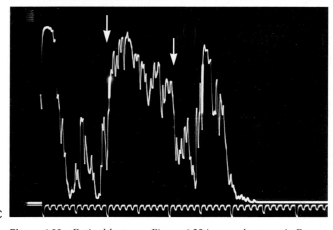

Figure 6.23 Retinoblastoma. Figure 6.23A: a moderate-gain B-scan showing a large, endophytic intraocular tumour. The lesion, owing to its high calcium content, is highly reflective and produces a shadowing effect (arrow). Figure 6.23B: a low-gain scan of the same lesion. Multiple calcium foci are better highlighted. Figure 6.23C: A-scan at T-sensitivity. The tumour shows high-amplitude echoes (between arrows) and the orbital spikes are reduced because of shadowing

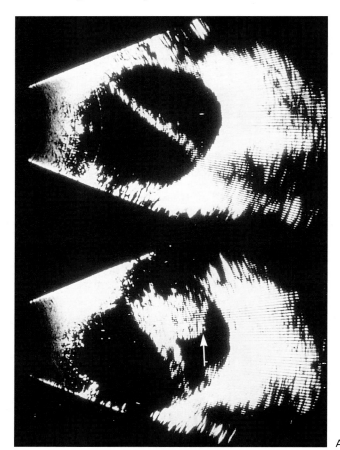

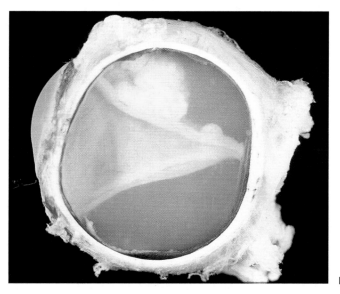

Figure 6.24 An exophytic retinoblastoma. Figure 6.24A: B-scans demonstrating an extensive retinal detachment and a large tumour mass in the subretinal space (arrow). Figure 6.24B: the echographic findings are confirmed on macroscopic examination of the enucleated eye (courtesy of S. F. Byrne)

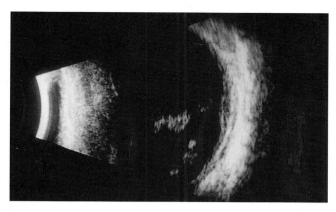 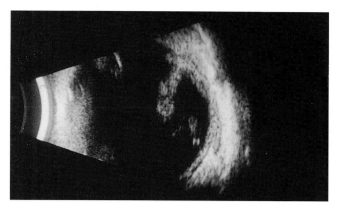

Figure 6.25 Atypical form of retinoblastoma presenting as mild thickening of the retino-choroid layer and non-specific vitreous opacities. Calcification was not detected

Careful scanning of the entire globe, retrobulbar optic nerve, and orbital fat is essential, using high and low gain settings. In many cases examination without anaesthesia or with mild sedation is adequate. General anaesthesia, however, may still be indicated in some children to allow thorough and complete examination.

Important features to observe during the dynamic scanning include the presence of calcification (and shadowing), vascularity, retinal detachment and cysts,

cyclitic or retrolental membranes, prominence of the ciliary body, vitreous cells and strands or bands, sub-retinal cholesterol deposits, optic nerve enlargement, orbital mass, and asymmetry of the axial eye length.

Retinoblastoma is characterized by the presence of a solid mass lesion exhibiting various degrees of vascularity (as seen on A-scan). Calcification within the lesion is a diagnostic feature (Figure 6.23).[10,11] This may be marked, producing a single highly reflective

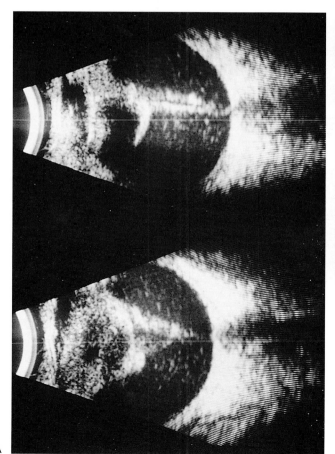

A

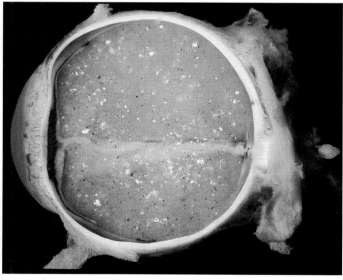

B

Figure 6.26 Advanced Coats' disease. Figure 6.26A: at the top, a vertical axial scan showing a closed-funnel retinal detachment, anchored to the optic nerve. At the bottom, a horizontal axial section; the retinal funnel is more open. In both sections, the subretinal space is filled with dense dispersed opacities representing cholesterol deposits. Figure 6.26B: the pathological appearance of the enucleated eye shows massive subretinal exudates dotted with shiny cholesterol crystals, and the detached retina appears as a line (closed funnel) (courtesy of Dr G. Scott)

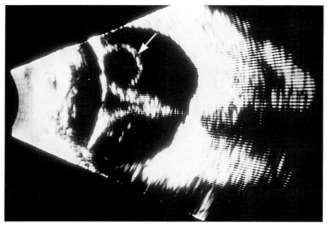

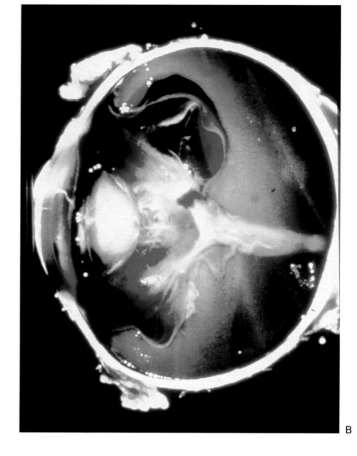

Figure 6.27 Advanced retinopathy of prematurity (ROP). Figure 6.27A: the scan shows a total, narrow-funnel retinal detachment adherent to the back of the lens, where a large peripheral subretinal cyst (arrow) is seen. The subretinal space is relatively clear. Figure 6.27B: the macroscopic appearance of the enucleated eye confirms the echographic findings (courtesy of S. F. Byrne)

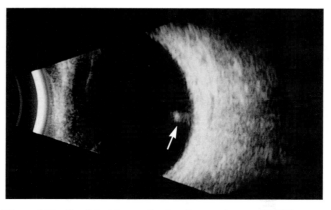

Figure 6.28 Persistent hyperplastic primary vitreous (PHPV). Figure 6.28A: a longitudinal scan showing a linear, cord-like opacity extending from the optic nerve head to the fundus periphery. Note the prominence of the ciliary body (arrow). Figure 6.28B: a transverse section taken at right angles to the previous scan. A cross-section of the 'cord' opacity is demonstrated (arrow)

coalescent plaque(s) with shadowing effect, or multiple small refractile spots, dispersed throughout the tumour mass. These are best seen at low gain settings. Retinal detachment may be associated with retinoblastoma, particularly in the exophytic type (Figure 6.24), and small tumour seedlings may be seen along retinal surfaces and in the vitreous. Careful scanning of the optic nerve and adjacent orbital fat is essential to exclude extraocular extension of tumour. Scanning of the other eye should also be performed to detect bilateral disease. The axial length in retinoblastoma is normal, or slightly increased in some uniocular cases.

Atypical forms of retinoblastoma may occasionally be encountered and are often difficult to diagnose.[12,13,14,15] Some tumours appear on echography as mild, diffuse thickening of the retino-choroid layer, with or without vitreous infiltration (Figure 6.25). Absence of calcification has been reported in a number of cases.[12,13,15] This is likely to occur in the early stages of the disease and in the diffuse type. Frequent follow-up studies are essential in such circumstances to document any increase in diameters and detect early calcification.

Coats' disease presents as a unilateral exudative retinal detachment with characteristically dense, mobile, subretinal deposits made of cholesterol crystals (Figure 6.26).[8,16] The vitreous cavity usually remains clear, and peripheral retinal loops may be seen. The axial eye length is normal.

Retinopathy of prematurity is normally a bilateral disease, but can be asymmetrical. Various stages of retinal detachment are seen, with peripheral loops or cysts in the advanced stages (Figure 6.27).[9,17] Subretinal opacities may be detected but they are not as pronounced as in Coats' disease. Vitreous and retrolental opacities are, however, common. The axial eye length is normal, but is reported to be shortened in severe cases.[9]

Persistent hyperplastic primary vitreous (PHPV) is typically a unilateral disease. The globe is shortened and the ciliary body becomes prominent as compared to the fellow eye. Characteristic single or multiple bands or cords are seen stretching from the optic disc to the posterior lens surface and also to the anterior periphery of the globe (Figure 6.28), where they occasionally produce limited tractional retinal detachment.

Table 6.1 summarizes the echographic features of common causes of leukokoria.

Table 6.1 Echographic diagnosis of leukokoria

Retinoblastoma	Coats' disease	ROP*	PHPV†
Unilateral/ bilateral	Unilateral	Bilateral	Unilateral
Solid mass	Retinal detachment	Retinal detachment	Band(s)
Calcification	Subretinal opacities	Retinal loops	Prominent ciliary body
Normal axial length	Normal axial length	Normal or short axial length	Short axial length

*ROP = retinopathy of prematurity.
†PHPV = persistent hyperplastic primary vitreous.

Anterior segment opacity

Ultrasonography is indicated in some cases of dense corneal opacities, especially when keratoplasty is being considered (Figure 6.29), and in chronic anterior uveitis with posterior synechia, where it is used to detect chorio-retinal thickening, macular oedema (Figure 6.30), choroidal effusion, cyclitic membrane,

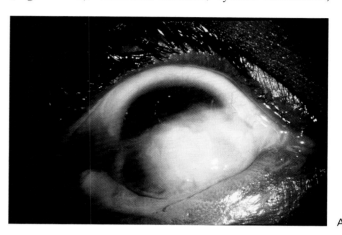
A

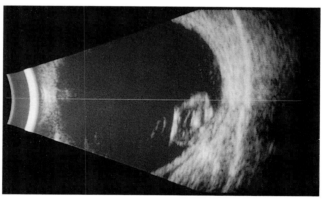
B

Figure 6.29 Figure 6.29A: the external appearance of an eye before undergoing penetrating keratoplasty. A dense corneal scar obstructed the view of the anterior segment and fundus.
Figure 6.29B: a B-scan showed that a cataractous lens had dislocated into the posterior segment, rendering the eye aphakic. This finding is likely to alter the surgical approach

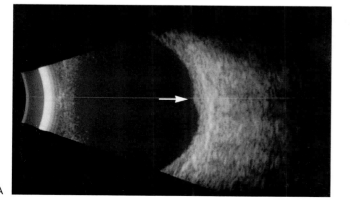
A

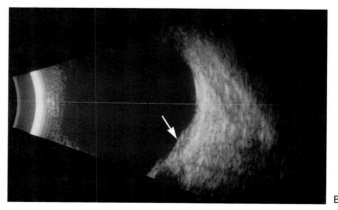
B

Figure 6.30 Transverse (Figure 6.30A) and longitudinal (Figure 6.30B) B-scans showing a mild, dome-shaped macular thickening (arrow) produced by macular oedema in a case of chronic pars planitis.

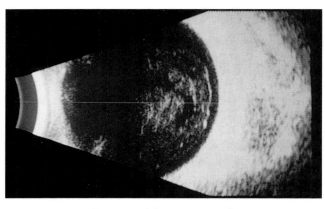

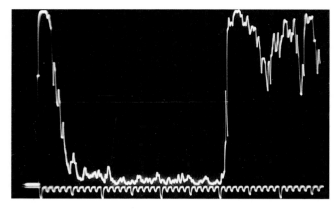

Figure 6.31 B- and A-scans of chronic uveitis, showing a moderate degree of vitreous opacities (cells). Fundoscopy may be hampered in such cases by posterior synechia or a cataract

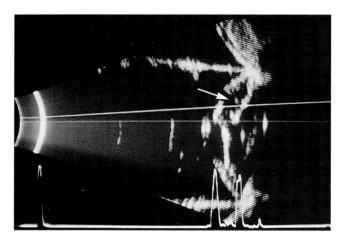

Figure 6.32 Immersion B-scan of an iris cyst (arrow)

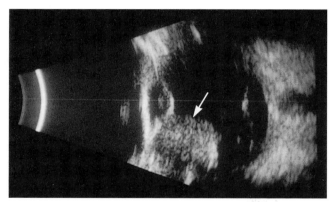

Figure 6.33 Immersion (vertical axial) B-scan showing a large, solid, inferior ciliary body mass in contact with the lens (arrow)

and vitreous opacities (cells) (Figure 6.31). In such cases, echography is likely to be a more accurate and objective method than the 'BIO scoring system',[18] which employs the indirect ophthalmoscope. In endophthalmitis cases, ultrasound is utilized to assess the degree of vitreous involvement and the effect of treatment.

In the above cases and in suspected iris and ciliary body cysts and tumours, the use of an immersion technique may prove superior for visualizing the anterior segment, iris/lens diaphragm, and anterior portion of the vitreous cavity (Figures 6.32, 6.33).

Blind painful eye

As ophthalmoscopy is often hampered in cases of blind painful eyes, ultrasound examination becomes necessary to evaluate the posterior segment. If visualization of the anterior segment is also obscured, immersion ultrasound technique is the method of choice.

The most important lesion to rule out is an uveal melanoma. Other findings may include 'chronic' reti-

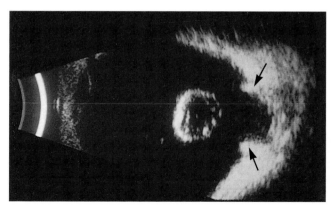

Figure 6.34 Dislocated, cataractous lens lying in the posterior vitreous. Note the apparent punched-out outline of the posterior globe wall and the 'Baum's bumps' (arrows). These are artefacts produced by a marked attenuation and scattering of sound waves as they travel through the lens

nal detachment, subretinal cysts (Figure 4.25), optic disc cupping (Figure 6.1), dislocated lens (Figure 6.34), and calcification of the retina and choroid. Massive disorganization and calcium deposition in the globe,

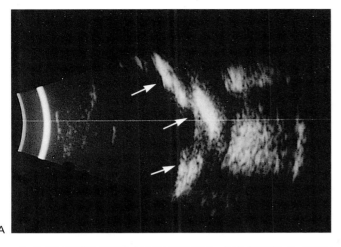

A

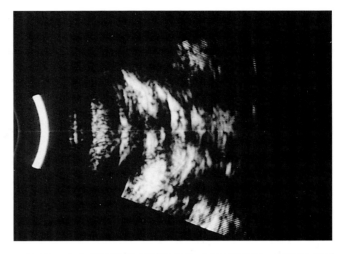

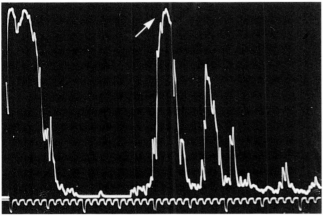

B

Figure 6.35 Intraocular calcification in a long-standing retinal detachment. On B-scan (Figure 6.35A), the retina is grossly thickened and is highly reflective with shadowing effect (arrows). On A-scan (Figure 6.35B) the retinal spike is thickened and tall (arrow), and the orbital spikes are weakened because of shadowing

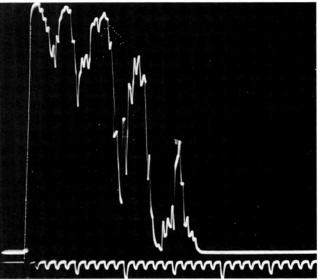

Figure 6.36 Intraocular calcification in a phthisical eye. No recognizable anatomy is seen on B- or A-scan. Instead, the intraocular contents are replaced by a disorganized calcified mass

with occasional bone formation, are frequent findings in phthisis bulbi and in eyes with previous blunt trauma and failed retinal detachment surgery (Figures 6.35, 6.36)

CLEAR MEDIA

Intraocular tumours

Echography is a very useful tool in the detection, differentiation, and measurement of intraocular tumours. The echographic features of choroid melanoma, metastasis, and choroidal haemangioma have already been described in Chapter 4.

Echographic examination may add to the clinical findings, even if the lesion is clearly seen on ophthalmoscopy. For instance, in melanoma an extrascleral extension (Figure 4.45) may be detected. This is an important prognostic sign, unlikely to have been noted on fundoscopy. Echography is also helpful in the 'work-up' of patients undergoing radiotherapy, since it provides accurate localization and measurements of the lesion. Tumours treated with radiotherapy exhibit an alteration in their internal structure and reflectivity (on A-scan), presumably due to the resultant necrosis and fibrosis within the tumour (Figure 4.47).[19,20]

Other fundus lesions

Choroidal nevus is either flat (not detected) or slightly thickened on echography. Quantitative A-scan examination may be difficult to undertake as the height of these lesions is often insufficient. However, nevi are predominantly high in reflectivity (Figure 6.37). An

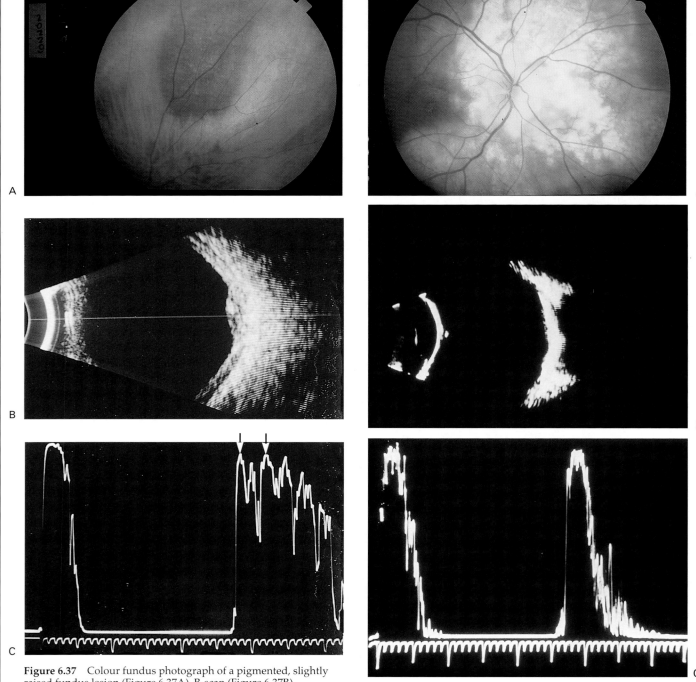

Figure 6.37 Colour fundus photograph of a pigmented, slightly raised fundus lesion (Figure 6.37A). B-scan (Figure 6.37B) confirmed a slight dome-shaped elevation. A-scan (Figure 6.37C) shows a highly reflective pattern (between arrows) consistent with a benign nevus. Follow-up studies of such a lesion are important to detect growth and change (reduction) in reflectivity; both are signs of malignant transformation

Figure 6.38 Choroidal osteoma. Colour photograph (Figure 6.38A) and B- and A-scans (Figures 6.38B and 6.38C). Owing to the lesion's high calcium content, the involved segment of the globe wall is highly reflective and orbital echoes are greatly reduced because of shadowing (courtesy of S. F. Byrne)

increase in height and reduction in reflectivity on follow-up studies should raise the suspicion of a malignant transformation.[21]

Choroidal osteoma, owing to its high calcium content, produces a spectacular appearance, whereby the involved segment becomes highly reflective – with or without detectable thickening of the choroid – and produces a large shadowing effect, blocking the orbital echoes posterior to the lesion (Figure 6.38).

Posterior scleritis appears as an area of low reflectivity between the outer sclera and orbital fat (Tenon's space), with associated thickening of the 'globe wall'

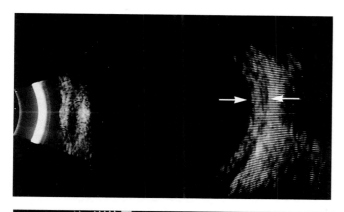

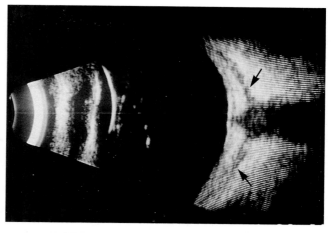

A

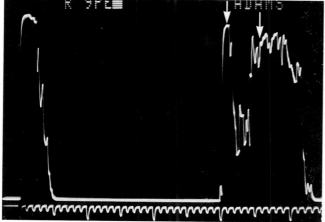

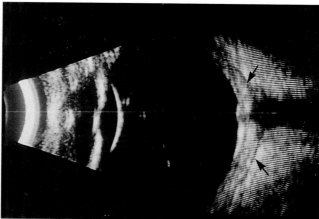

B

Figure 6.39 Posterior scleritis: transverse B- and A-scans of the equatorial region showing low-reflective thickening of the globe wall (arrows), probably the result of oedema and infiltration of the Tenon's or episcleral space

Figure 6.40 Vertical (Figure 6.40A) and horizontal (Figure 6.40B) axial scans of posterior scleritis. As the inflammation spreads along the Tenon's space (arrow) back to the optic nerve sheaths, a characteristic 'T-sign' is produced

(Figure 6.39). Spreading of the inflammatory process to the optic nerve's sheaths gives rise to the so-called 'T-sign' (Figure 6.40).

Choroidal folds, one of the signs of posterior scleritis, is an indication for ultrasound examination.[22] Some folds are idiopathic with no apparent cause. In such cases shortening of the axial length and progressive hypermetropia are observed.

Choroidal folds are also produced by an orbital-space-occupying lesion. This will be discussed in Chapter 9.

OCULAR TRAUMA

Echography is required in many cases of blunt and sharp ocular trauma, and in the detection and management of intraocular foreign bodies.

In blunt trauma, fundoscopy may be hampered by pupillary abnormality and poor dilatation, Descemet's folds, hyphaema, traumatic cataract, and vitreous haemorrhage. Echography supplies information on the state of the lens – e.g. rupture or dislocation (Figures 6.29, 6.34, 6.41) – the presence and extent of vitreous haemorrhage and retinal detachment, and the presence of choroidal detachment and haemorrhage (Figure 6.42).

Posterior scleral rupture is suspected when a track of vitreous haemorrhage is seen incarcerating into a focal area at the posterior globe wall where the contour becomes irregular (Figures 6.43, 6.44). A low reflective area in the adjacent orbital fat is commonly found, representing a pocket of retrobulbar haemorrhage.

In blunt trauma with vitreous haemorrhage and poor fundus view, repeat echographic studies are helpful in assessing the need for, and timing of, vitrectomy through their detection of early retinal detachment, the development of posterior vitreous detachment, and the presence and location of choroidal detachment and haemorrhage.

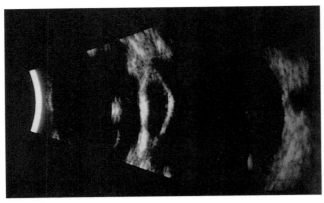
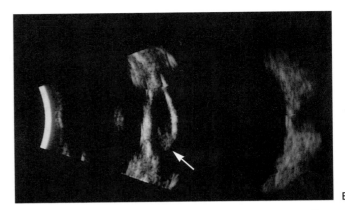

Figure 6.41 Traumatic rupture of the posterior lens surface. Immersion scans of the normal (Figure 6.41A) and traumatized (Figure 6.41B) eye. Compare the even curve of the normal posterior lens surface with the interrupted curve in the traumatized lens (arrow), at which point echoes within the lens are seen, indicating cataract formation

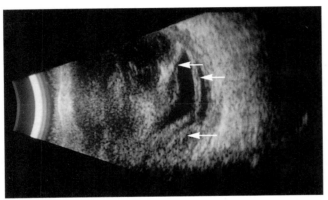
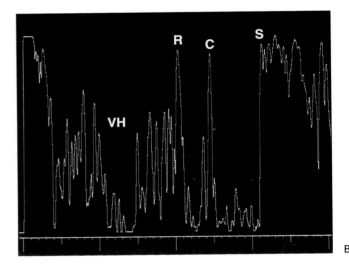

Figure 6.42 Blunt ocular trauma. Figure 6.42A: B-scan showing dense vitreous haemorrhage and PVD (top arrow), and retinal detachment (middle arrow) overlaying a haemorrhagic choroidal detachment (bottom arrow). Figure 6.42B: A-scan. Spikes of vitreous haemorrhage (VH) are followed by the high retinal spike (R) and choroidal detachment (C). A group of low-reflective echoes are seen between choroid and sclera (S), indicating supra-choroidal haemorrhage

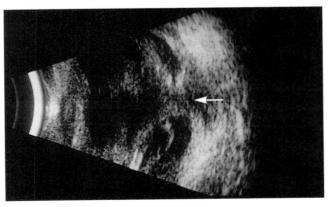
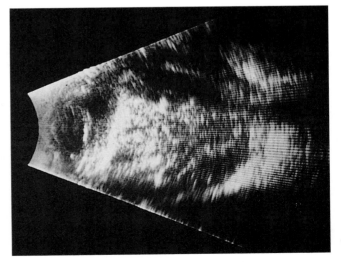

Figure 6.43 Posterior scleral rupture. The arrow points to the region of scleral rupture, where the (haemorrhagic) vitreous appears to adhere to an irregular and thickened segment of the globe wall. Note also the low-reflective zone in the adjacent orbit produced by a pocket of orbital haemorrhage

Figure 6.44 Posterior scleral rupture. The scan shows a dense vitreous haemorrhage, a vitreous track, and a low-reflective orbital haemorrhage behind scleral rupture

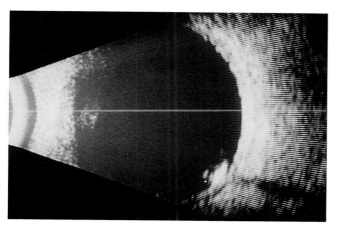

Figure 6.45 Intraocular foreign body (FB) seen in the inferior vitreous, adjacent to the retina. Note the characteristic shadowing effect. This FB was radiotranslucent and was not detected on plain X-ray

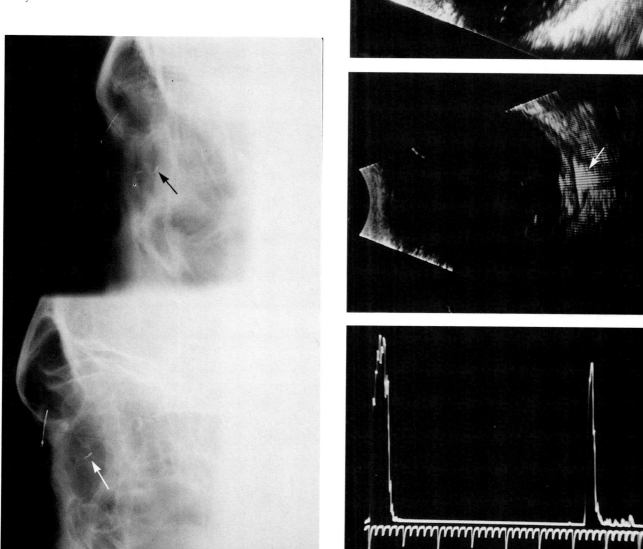

Figure 6.46 Figure 6.46A: lateral X-ray showing a linear radio-opaque opacity within the orbit (arrow), taken while the patient was looking up (top), and at primary gaze (bottom). No significant shift of FB was noted upon eye movements. A high-gain B-scan (Figure 6.46B) showed a posterior vitreous haemorrhage, and a low-gain scan (Figure 6.46C) detected the presence of a FB, which appears to be embedded in the globe wall (arrow). A-scan measurement of the axial distance of the FB signal (Figure 6.46D) confirmed its 'intramural' position

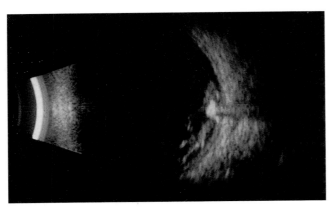

Figure 6.47 Intra-vitreal FB. The scan shows a high-reflective signal from a FB and shadowing with a surrounding vitreous haemorrhage. Kinetic examination revealed a free floating FB not attached to the globe wall

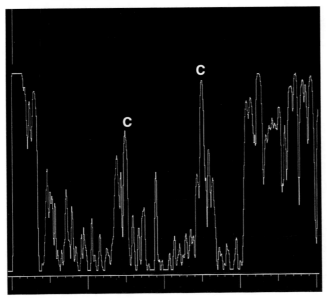

Figure 6.48 Expulsive haemorrhage. The B-scan (Figure 6.48A) demonstrates high (kissing) haemorrhagic choroidal detachments, totally occupying the vitreous space. The A-scan (Figure 6.48B) shows irregular haemorrhage spikes intercepted by tall choroidal spikes

In penetrating trauma, echography plays a lesser role, but may demonstrate lens rupture, posterior segment involvement, and a retained foreign body. Care must be taken to exert the least possible pressure on the globe and prevent infection. Examination through closed eyelids is therefore advisable in such cases.

Intraocular foreign bodies (FB) may only be detected on echography if they are radiotranslucent (Figure 6.45). Magnetic resonance imaging is generally not recommended in such cases.

In addition to the detection and localization of FB, concurrent damage to ocular tissues can be evaluated. Topographic and kinetic echography will show if the FB is adherent to or embedded in the retina (Figure 6.46), or if it is floating in the vitreous (Figure 6.47). In the former case, vitrectomy and direct instrumental removal of FB is considered safer than magnet removal. Repeat ultrasound examination is recommended after extraction of FB to exclude retained particles.

Traumatic complications of ocular surgery include expulsive haemorrhage (Figure 6.48), which may be

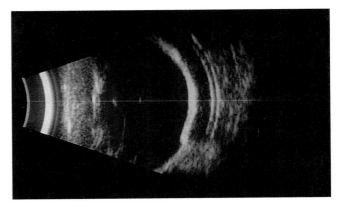

Figure 6.49 B-scan echogram of a circumferential scleral buckle. The low-reflective C-shaped orbital opacity is produced by the shadowing effect of the explant

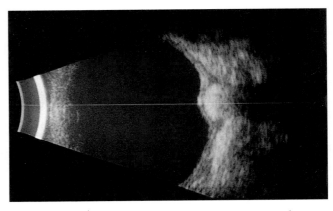

Figure 6.50 Transverse B-scan of a radial scleral sponge. The retina follows the contour of the indent with no evidence of subretinal fluid

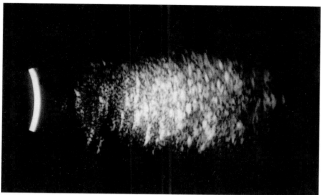

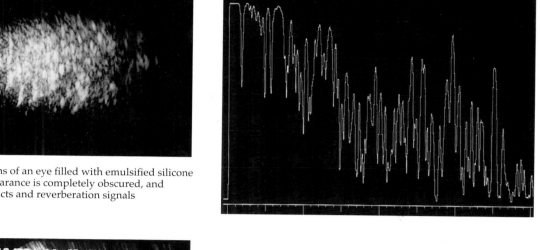

Figure 6.51 A- and B-scans of an eye filled with emulsified silicone oil. The normal globe appearance is completely obscured, and replaced by multiple artefacts and reverberation signals

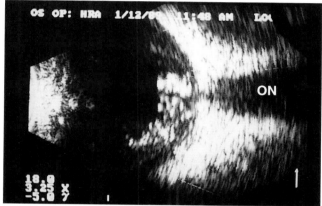

Figure 6.52 Retained heavy liquid (perfluorodecalin). Multiple, highly reflective liquid bubbles are seen in the posterior vitreous space. Interestingly, no shadowing effect was detected behind the bubbles. ON = optic nerve

delayed.[23] In eyes with previous retinal detachment and vitrectomy surgery, echography may show the scleral explant (Figures 6.49, 6.50). The ultrasound image may be altered or obscured by residual gas/air, emulsified silicone oil (Figure 6.51), and retained heavy liquid (Figure 6.52).

REFERENCES

1 Byrne S F. Differential diagnosis of disciform lesions using standardized echography. In: Hillman J S, LeMay M M (eds) Ophthalmic ultrasound. Dordrecht: Junk, 1983:149–162

2 Cunliffe I A, Rennie I G. Choroidal melanoma presenting as vitreous haemorrhage. Eye 1993; 7:711–713

3 Butner R W, McPherson A R. Spontaneous vitreous hemorrhage. Ann Ophthalmol 1982; 14:268–270

4 Green R L. The echographic evaluation of spontaneous vitreous hemorrhage. In: Ossoinig K C (ed) Ophthalmic echography. Doc Ophthalmol Proc Ser 1987; 48:233–238

5 Bosanquet R C, Bell J A. Is B-scan ultrasound useful in predicting the source of vitreous hemorrhage? In: Till P (ed) Ophthalmic echography. Dordrecht; Kluwer, 1993:333–336

6 Ossoinig K C. Echographic detection and classification of posterior hyphemas. Ophthalmologica 1984; 189:2–11

7 Byrne S F, Green R L. Ultrasound of the eye and orbit. St Louis: Mosby Year Book, 1992:60–61

8 Atta H R, Watson N J. Echographic diagnosis of advanced Coats' disease. Eye 1992; 6:80–85

9 Pulido J S, Byrne S F, Clarkson J G et al. Evaluation of eyes with advanced stages of retinopathy of prematurity using standardized echography. Ophthalmology 1991; 98:1099–1104

10 Ossoinig K C, Cennamo G, Green R L et al. Echographic results in the diagnosis of retinoblastoma. In: Thijssen J M, Verbeek A M (eds) Ultrasonography in ophthalmology. Dordrecht: Junk, 1981; 29:103–107

11 Sterns G K, Coleman D J, Ellsworth R M. The ultrasonographic characteristics of retinoblastoma. Am J Ophthalmol 1974; 78:606–611

12 Nicholson D H, Norton E W D. Diffuse infiltrating retinoblastoma. Tr Am Ophthalmol Soc 1980; 78:265–289

13 Schofield P B. Diffuse infultrating retinoblastoma. Br J Ophthalmol 1960; 44:35–41

14 Soll D B, Turtz A I. Retinoblastoma diagnosed as granulomatous uveitis. Arch Ophthalmol 1960; 63:687–691

15 Lombardi A, Irarrazaval L A, Croxatto J O et al. Ultrasonographic findings in selected cases of masquerading syndrome. In: Sampaolesi (ed) Ultrasonography in ophthalmology. Dordrecht: Kluwer, 1990:313–319

16 Haik B G, Smith M E, Ellsworth R M et al. Ultrasonography in the diagnosis of advanced Coats' disease. In: Ossoinig K C (ed) Ophthalmic echography. Dordrecht: Junk, 1987:428

17 Patz A, Palmer E A. Retinopathy of prematurity. In: Ryan S J (ed) Retina, vol 2. St Louis: Mosby, 1989

18 BenEzra D, Forrester J V, Nussenblatt R B et al. Uveitis scoring system. Berlin: Springer-Verlag, 1991

19 Saornil M A, Egan K M, Gragoudas E S et al. Histopathology of proton beam-irradiated vs. enucleated uveal melanomas. Arch Ophthalmol 1992; 110:1112–1118

20 Gragoudas E S, Egan K M, Saornil M A et al. The time course of irradiation changes in proton beam-treated uveal melanomas. Ophthalmology 1993; 100:1555–1559

21 Ossoinig K C, Lohmeyer M. Choroidal nevi: diagnosis with standardized echography. In: Sampaolesi (ed) Ultrasonography in ophthalmology. Dordrecht: Kluwer, 1990

22 Atta H R, Byrne S F. The findings of standardized echography for choroidal folds. Arch Ophthalmol 1988; 106:1234–1241

23 Hoffman P, Pollack A, Oliver M. Limited choroidal haemorrhage associated with intracapsular cataract extraction. Arch Ophthalmol 1984; 102:1761–1765

THE ORBIT

7

Orbital screening

The successful detection and classification of orbital lesions depends on a rigorous routine of screening, and on summation of the maximum possible acoustic data, many of which are derived from standardized A-scan, supported by B-scan and Doppler ultrasound.[1,2] More so than in the globe, repeated comparison between the two orbits is essential to detect subtle abnormalities and document bilateral disease – a common feature of orbital abnormalities. Table 7.1 summarizes the spectrum of acoustic information and the scanning mode best used to obtain it.

In contrast to the globe, the orbit is predominantly high reflective, owing to heterogeneity of the orbital fat which produces large acoustic interfaces (Figure 7.1).

Other normal structures and most of the abnormal lesions in the orbit are usually less reflective, because of their more regular tissue arrangement. They appear, therefore, as a defect on A-scan and a dark outline on B-scan (Figure 7.2).

Table 7.1 Orbital echography: acoustic data and preferred scanning mode	
Data	**Scanning mode**
Screening	
Orbital fat	A and B
Optic nerve	A
Extraocular muscles	A and B
Lacrimal gland	A and B
Bony orbit and sinuses	B and A
Topographic examination	
Shape	B
Borders	A and B
Location	B and A
Quantitative echography	
Reflectivity	A and B
Internal structure or texture	A
Sound attenuation	A
Kinetic echography	
Consistency	A and B
Vascularity	A and Doppler
Valsalva test	B and A
30° test	A

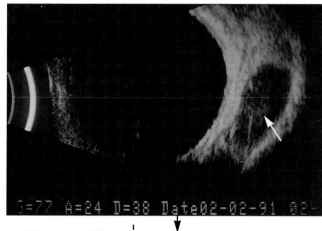

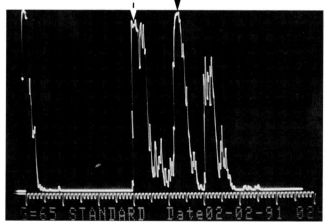

Figure 7.2 Abnormal orbital scan. On B-scan (Figure 7.2A) this appears as a dark outline (arrow) and on A-scan (Figure 7.2B) as a defect (between two arrows)

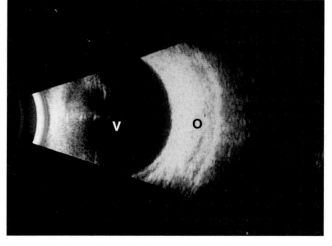

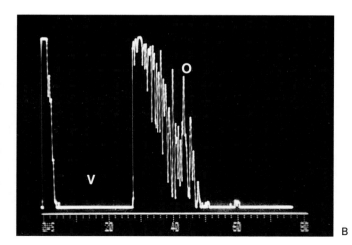

Figure 7.1 Normal orbital echogram. Unlike the globe with its anechoic vitreous cavity (V), the orbit (O) is highly reflective due to heterogeneity of the orbital fat. On B-scan (Figure 7.1A) this appears as a bright zone, and on A-scan (Figure 7.1B) as tightly packed, tall spikes that fade rapidly from left to right

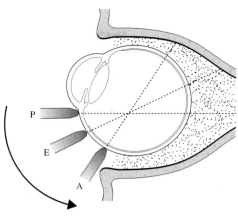

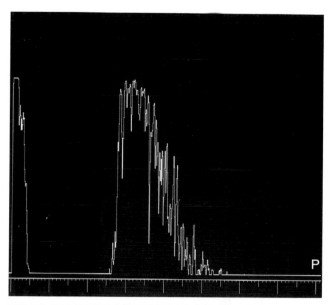

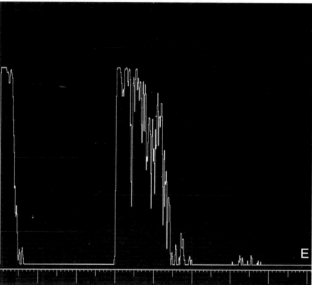

Figure 7.3 Transocular A-scan. Line drawing illustrating probe position and beam orientation in posterior (P), equator (E), and anterior (A) sections. In the actual echograms, note the reduction in width of the fat segment as the beam is shifted more anteriorly. Also, as the beam is oriented more perpendicularly against the orbital wall in the anterior (A) section (bottom), a high amplitude 'bone spike' develops (arrow)

Most of the ultrasound instruments used in ophthalmology do not permit adequate visualization of the orbital apex. This is the result of a compromise between resolution and penetration of sound waves. Resolution is enhanced by increasing the frequency of sound, which in turn reduces the ability of ultrasonic waves to scan adequately the deeper tissues. However, lesions in this 'crowded' area invariably produce a 'mass effect', giving rise to venous obstruction, distension of the optic nerve sheaths, and other findings readily detected during scanning of the anterior orbital compartment.

Complete orbital screening involves examination of the following:

1. Orbital fat.
2. Extraocular muscles.
3. Optic nerve.
4. Lacrimal gland.
5. Bony walls and periorbita.

The general preparation of instruments and patient is similar to that described for ocular screening in Chapters 2 and 3.

ORBITAL FAT SCREENING

Screening of the orbital fat is performed to detect mass lesions, foreign bodies, haemorrhage, cellulitis, distension of orbital vessels, and general increase in fat volume.

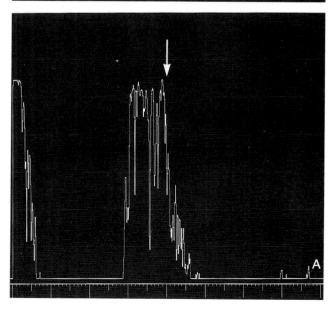

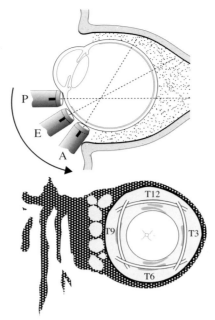

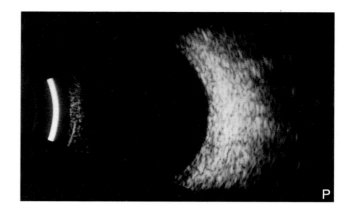

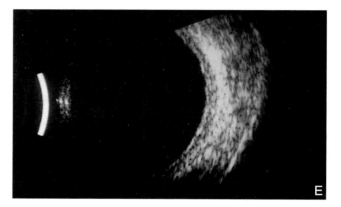

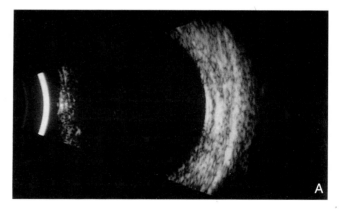

Figure 7.4 Transocular transverse B-scan. Above: two line drawings illustrating the probe position and beam orientation in relation to orbital structures. Left: the echograms. P = posterior, E = equator, A = anterior sections. As in the A-scan, the orbital fat segment is reduced in width as the beam is shifted anteriorly

Two approaches are available: transocular and paraocular. The former (through the globe) is employed to detect lesions located posterior to the equatorial plane of the eye, while the latter (avoiding the globe) is suitable for scanning anteriorly placed lesions such as lacrimal gland tumours, mucoceles, and dermoid cysts. Both approaches can be performed with A- and B-scan.

Transocular A-scan screening (Figure 7.3)

The instrument is set at tissue sensitivity. Eight meridians are scanned antero-posteriorly as in ocular screening. In addition, examination of the corresponding meridians in the opposite orbit is performed for comparison. The normal orbital fat appears as a highly reflective, tightly packed group of spikes, commencing immediately to the right of the scleral signal, and fading rapidly from left to right. This is due to strong sound attenuation. The width of the 'fat segment' on A-scan is greatest when the probe is directed axially towards the orbital apex and narrowest when the beam is tilted towards the anterior orbital compartment (Figure 7.3). Orbital fat spikes also exhibit unique fast oscillation, distinguishing them from the much slower spikes of abnormal lesions.

The examiner therefore observes the orbital segment of the echogram for abnormal widening of the fat, development of a defect in the pattern, and slowing down in the oscillation of spikes. This task is made easier if one compares the two orbits.

Transocular B-scan screening

Four transverse sections (T-12, T-3, T-6, and T-9 o'clock hours), are performed in a manner similar to that described for ocular screening, using medium to low decibel gain (Figure 7.4). Vertical and horizontal axial sections are also obtained to demonstrate the lesion's relation to the optic nerve (Figure 7.5).

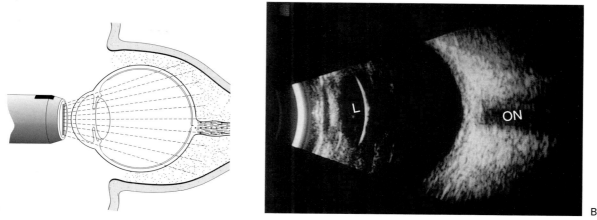

Figure 7.5 Axial B-scan of the orbit taken to demonstrate the relation of lesions to the optic nerve. L = lens, ON = optic nerve

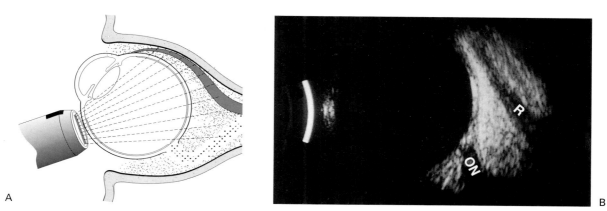

Figure 7.6 Longitudinal B-scan of the orbit, employed to demonstrate the relation of lesions to rectus muscle (R) and optic nerve (ON). Also helpful in determining whether a lesion is extra- or intra-conal

Longitudinal and other transverse and axial sections may additionally be carried out, depending on the location of the lesion, for accurate localization and documentation.

The normal orbit appears as a homogeneous bright zone, and, depending on the beam location, the dark outline of the optic nerve and extraocular muscles may be seen (Figure 7.6).

Paraocular A- and B-scanning (Figure 7.7)

Both modes can be used to scan the anterior orbital compartment, including the preseptal space. This is performed by applying liberal amounts of coupling jelly to the closed eyelids and placing the probe firmly in the space between globe and orbital rim. As the beam is shifted away from the globe, the orbital fat pattern appears immediately following the initial spike. Screening of all meridians is performed with A-Scan, including comparison with the other orbit. Transverse and longitudinal B-scan sections of suspected areas are also carried out. In addition, 'stand-off' technique may be employed to identify anterior paraocular lesions. To maintain standardization of A-scan, 3 decibels are added to the T-sensitivity gain to compensate for energy absorbed through the skin.

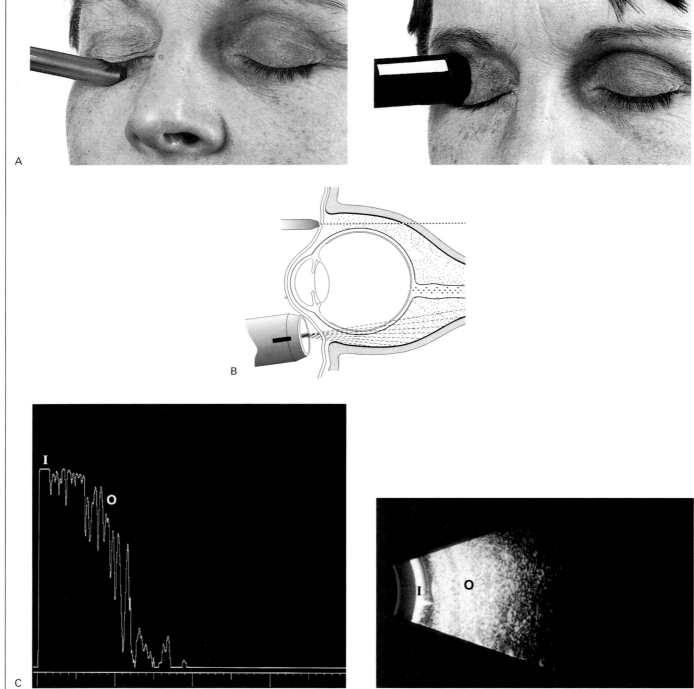

Figure 7.7 Paraocular screening of orbital fat. Figure 7.7A: the probe is placed on the skin, near the orbital margin. Figure 7.7B: line drawing illustrating probe position and beam orientation for A- and B-scans. Figure 7.7C: the resulting echograms. The initial signal (I) is immediately followed by the orbital fat (O)

EXAMINATION OF EXTRAOCULAR MUSCLES

The extraocular muscles, particularly the four recti, lend themselves well to ultrasound scanning because of their easily traced anatomical location and their regular histological structure.[3]

A cross sectional A-scan display of a rectus muscle appears as a defect in the orbital pattern, delineated by two tall, double-peaked, smoothly rising spikes originating from the muscle sheaths. The muscle proper appears as a medium-reflective group of spikes (Figure 7.8). Biometry of the muscle thickness is undertaken by measurement of the distance between the two opposing sides of the sheath spikes.

Transverse and longitudinal sections of the four recti are also obtained on B-scan (Figure 7.9), and appear as a dark (low-reflective) outline. The oblique muscles, owing to their diagonal course, are difficult to measure precisely on A-scan, but can be displayed on B-scan (Figure 7.10).

A-scan technique

The instrument is set at tissue sensitivity. As the muscle thickness alters during contraction and relaxation, it is essential to conduct scanning with the eyelids open and the patient gazing at the primary position. The probe is placed on the globe, opposite the muscle to be scanned; the beam is aimed at the opposite equa-

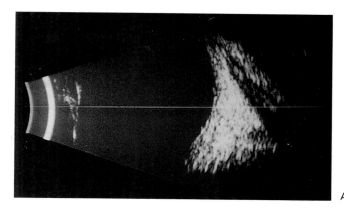

A

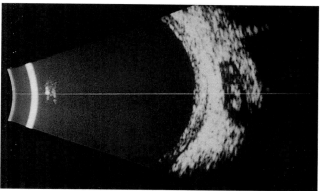

B

Figure 7.9 Normal B-scan of a rectus muscle. Figure 7.9A is a longitudinal display and Figure 7.9B a transverse display. The muscle is less reflective (darker) than the surrounding fat

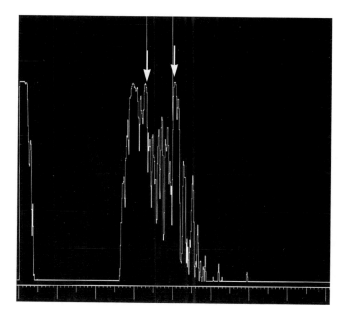

Figure 7.8 Normal A-scan trace of a rectus muscle. The muscle fibres are less reflective than the surrounding fat, and appear therefore as a defect of medium/medium-high reflectivity outlined by two steeply rising tall spikes from the muscle sheaths (arrows)

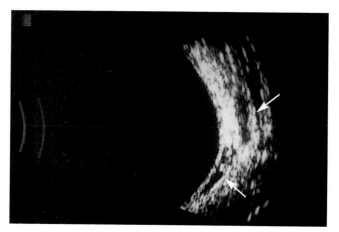

Figure 7.10 B-scan of inferior oblique muscle. The top arrow points at a transverse section of the inferior rectus, and the bottom arrow at the inferior oblique

103

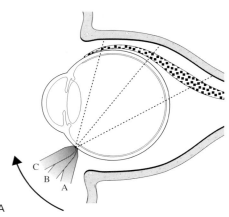

Figure 7.11 Technique of A-scanning of rectus muscles. Above: the probe is placed opposite the muscle to be scanned. Starting with the insertion (position A), the beam is swept posteriorly, scanning mid belly (position B) and posterior third (position C). Left: echograms A, B, and C are the corresponding traces for each of the probe positions. Note the widening of the muscle defect (arrow) as it shifts from left to right along the orbital fat

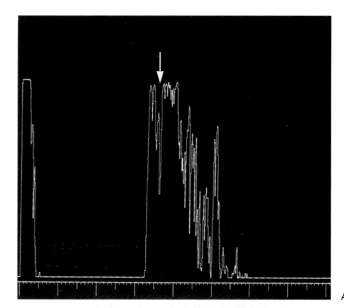

A

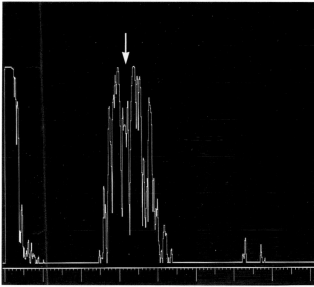

B

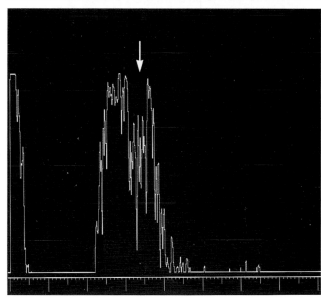

C

tor and swept posteriorly, scanning the muscle along its length, starting with the insertion (Figure 7.11). Fine adjustment of the probe position is undertaken until the best possible trace is obtained. Biometry of the muscle thickness is performed at its widest diameter, nearer the posterior third of the belly. Scanning of the two vertical recti may occasionally be difficult because of their slightly oblique course and, particularly in the case of the inferior rectus, prominence of the orbital rim. In addition, the superior rectus and levator muscle are normally inseparable on echography and are therefore measured as one unit. Recently published data on the range of normal muscle thickness[4] are presented in Table 7.2.

Table 7.2 Diameters of extraocular muscles in normal population (reproduced with permission from American Journal of Ophthalmology 112(6):710) 1991

Muscle	Mean	SD (mm)	Median
Superior rectus/ levator complex	5.3	0.7	5.4
Lateral rectus	3.0	0.4	3.1
Inferior rectus	2.6	0.5	2.6
Medial rectus	3.5	0.6	3.6
Sum of all muscles	14.4	1.3	14.6

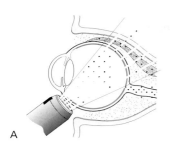

A

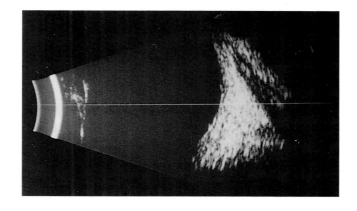

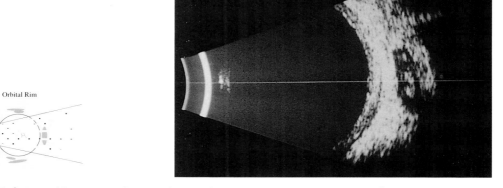

Orbital Rim

B

Figure 7.12 Technique of B-scanning of extraocular muscle. Figure 7.12A: line drawing and echogram illustrating longitudinal muscle section. The beam is aligned 'along' the muscle, scanning from its insertion to the posterior belly. Figure 7.12B: the transverse section. The beam is now scanning 'across' the muscle. In this illustration, the medial rectus muscle is examined

B-scan technique

A transverse (cross-section) and a longitudinal display of each of the four rectus muscles can be obtained on B-scan (Figure 7.12). This is best performed through the open eyelids using medium to medium/low decibel gain. The patient may gaze at the primary position or towards the muscle to be scanned for better alignment of the sound beam. The two horizontal recti are scanned by placing the probe at the opposite side of the globe, with its marker up for transverse sections, and at the limbus for longitudinal sections. The vertical recti are scanned by placing the probe on the opposite side, with the marker nasally for transverse and at the limbus for longitudinal sections. The oblique muscles are displayed during examination of the inferior rectus (inferior oblique) and superior rectus (superior oblique) (Figure 7.10).

OPTIC NERVE ECHOGRAPHY

The tubular structure of the optic nerve with its homogeneous, low-reflective, parallel nerve fibre bundle, surrounded by the distinctly high-reflective dural sheaths, makes the optic nerve an ideal structure for ultrasound imaging.[5,6,7]

A reliable biometry of the nerve thickness along its anterior two-thirds is performed with standardized A-scan which, through kinetic echography, can also differentiate between fluid sheath distension and solid nerve thickening (the 30° test) – a feature not readily available in other imaging techniques.

A-scan technique

The instrument is set at tissue sensitivity. The probe is firmly placed at the temporal equator, resting on the bony orbital rim, and the patient fixates at the primary position or slightly infra-temporally (Figure 7.13). The sound beam is directed postero-nasally and slightly up, and shifted towards the orbital apex, scanning the nerve antero-posteriorly. The examiner makes fine adjustments of the probe/eye position and observes the screen until a distinct defect appears in the orbital fat pattern adjacent to the scleral spike (Figure 7.14). Unlike the rectus muscles, the width of the defect does not alter significantly as the nerve is traced posteriorly; only the amplitude of the sheaths' spikes is reduced, owing to sound attenuation. The wider defect of the medial rectus muscle may occasionally appear next to, and should not be mistaken for, the nerve defect.

The author's figures for normal echographic width of the optic nerve range from 2.4 mm to 3.4 mm with a median of 2.9 mm and no more than 0.3 mm difference between the two nerves. Slightly different figures have been published by others.[5,7,8] This is likely to reflect inter-observer variation. Each observer, therefore, should derive his or her own figures for reliable interpretation of results.

The 30° test (Figure 7.15)

The unique feature of 'real time', dynamic ultrasound scanning is best illustrated by this test, which allows

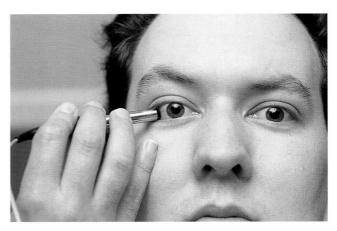

Figure 7.13 A-scan approach for optic nerve examination. Probe is aiming nasally, posteriorly, and slightly superiorly

the differentiation of fluid sheaths distension from solid nerve lesion as a cause of optic nerve swelling.[7,8]

A-scan measurement of the nerve width is obtained in the primary gaze as described above. The patient then abducts the eye approximately 30° and the measurement is repeated. Normally no alteration in the nerve measurement is obtained. If the nerve is widened from sheath distension, abduction of the eye results in stretching of the nerve, redistribution of the subarachnoid fluid within the sheaths, and a net reduction in the nerve width. If solid nerve thickening is present, however, no decrease, or even an increase,

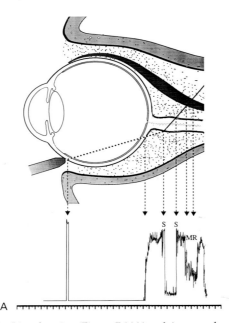

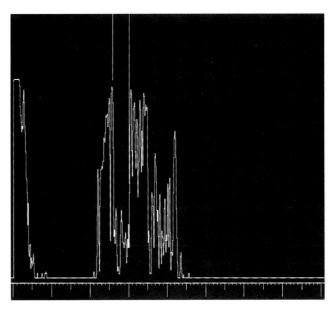

Figure 7.14 Line drawing (Figure 7.14A) and A-scan echogram (Figure 7.14B) of the optic nerve. The drawing illustrates the probe and beam orientation and the resulting trace. Favourable refraction of the sound beam at the fat/nerve sheath interfaces produces high-reflecting sheath spikes (S) on either side of the low-reflective nerve proper. Oblique incidence of the beam on the posterior globe wall and medial rectus (MR) results in a weak scleral signal and irregular muscle defect

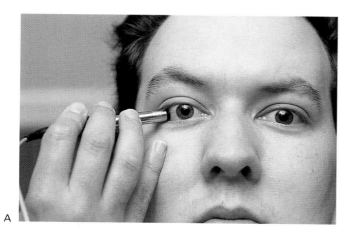

A

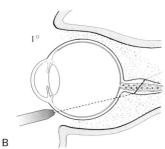

1°

B

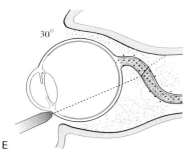

D

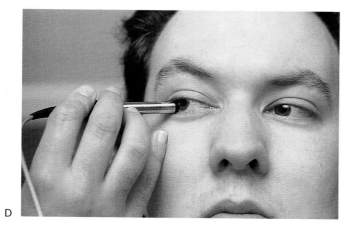

30°

E

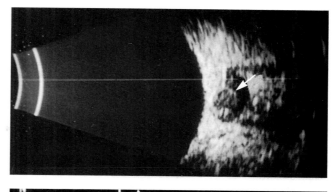

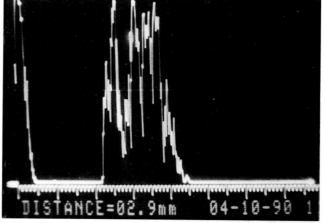

DISTANCE=02.9mm   04-10-90 1

C

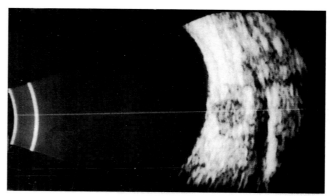

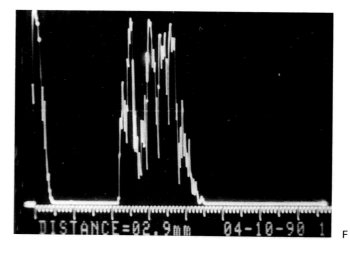

DISTANCE=02.9mm   04-10-90 1

F

Figure 7.15 The 30° test. Figure 7.15A: the probe/eye position in primary gaze. Figure 7.15B: line drawing of a distended nerve measured in primary gaze. Figure 7.15C: B- and A-scans showing distension of the nerve with a primary gaze measurement of 4.2 mm. Note that on the B-scan the nerve 'proper' can be seen adjacent to the distended subarachnoid space (arrow). Figure 7.15D: the probe/eye position in 30° of abduction. Figure 7.15E: the nerve is stretched and fluid redistributed. Figure 7.15F: B- and A-scans of nerve. Note the disappearance of 'fluid' on the B-scan and the reduction of the nerve measurement to 2.9 mm on the A-scan

in nerve diameter occurs. A reduction in nerve width of 10% or more is considered positive. The validity of this test has been proven in experimental studies and in patients undergoing surgical nerve sheath decompression.[9,10,11,12,13] Table 7.3 presents the causes of a positive and negative 30° test.

Table 7.3 Optic nerve swelling: causes of positive and negative 30° test	
Positive 30° test	Negative 30° test
Pseudotumour cerebri	Meningioma
Optic neuritis	Glioma
Trauma (blood)	Optic neuritis
Orbital venous congestion	
Choroidal effusion	Granuloma

B-scan technique of optic nerve scanning

The best echograms are obtained when the examination is conducted through open lids, using medium/low gain. A semi-quantitative assessment and comparison between the two nerves can be performed if the decibel gain and grey scale remain constant. B-mode scanning is also an ideal method for detecting optic disc abnormalities such as drüsen, coloboma, and oedema and for displaying calcification in the deeper portion of the nerve.

The optic nerve may be scanned via three approaches: axial, transverse, and longitudinal.

Axial section (Figure 7.16)

As the patient fixates at the primary position the probe is placed on the cornea and directed axially. The optic nerve appears as a tubular or a V-shaped dark outline – an obvious artefact probably produced by the marked sound scatter and reflection at the nerve head. This, in addition to the strong sound absorption by the lens, renders axial scanning unsuitable for displaying lesions in the deeper portion of the nerve.

Transverse section (Figure 7.17)

This section is useful for documenting widening of the anterior nerve portion and large optic nerve cupping. A cross-section of the nerve (salami cut) is produced by placing the probe temporally with the marker up. The beam, now oriented vertically, is directed posteronasally. The dark oval or round void of the nerve is displayed, located progressively away from the globe wall as the beam is swept towards the orbital apex. A more perpendicular display is obtained if the patient directs the gaze slightly towards the probe. A semi-quantitative assessment and comparison between the two eyes can be performed provided the decibel gain,

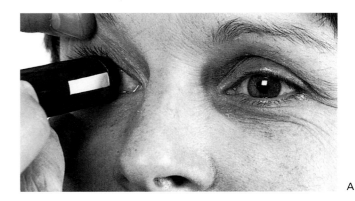

A

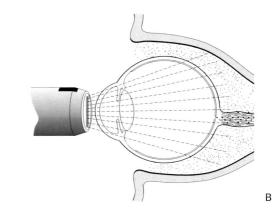

B

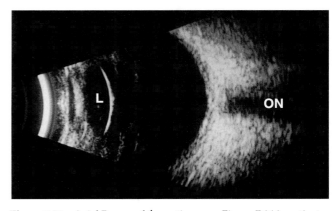

C

Figure 7.16 Axial B-scan of the optic nerve. Figure 7.16A: patient directs gaze at the primary position and the probe is placed axially on the cornea. Figure 7.16B: lens and nerve are centred in the beam. Figure 7.16C: posterior lens surface (L) and optic nerve (ON) are centred in the echogram. The V-shape appearance of the nerve is an obvious artefact, probably due to scatter and reflection of the sound beam at the nerve head

grey scale, and beam orientation remain constant. The 'crescent' and 'doughnut' signs described by Byrne and Green,[14] indicating nerve sheath distension, are best demonstrated on this section (Figure 7.18).

Longitudinal section (Figure 7.19)

As previously seen in ocular screening, all longitudinal sections display the optic nerve at the lower aspect

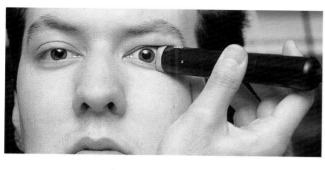

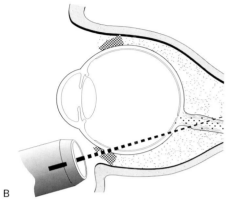

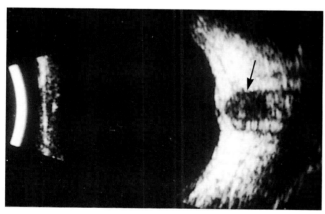

Figure 7.17 Transverse B-scan of the optic nerve. Figure 7.17A: the probe is placed temporally with its marker up. The patient directs gaze axially or slightly towards the probe. Figure 7.17B: line drawing of the probe/beam orientation. Figure 7.17C: the nerve appears as a dark, round, or oval void behind the globe wall (arrow). The distance between the void and globe increases as the nerve is traced posteriorly

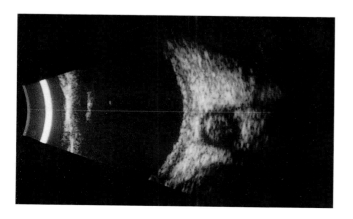

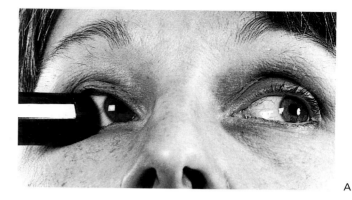

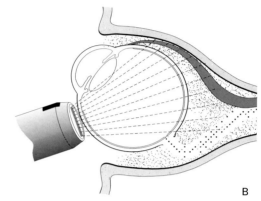

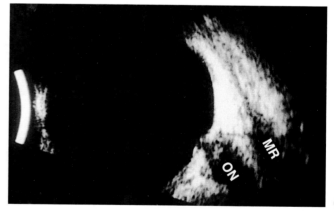

Figure 7.19 Longitudinal B-scan of the optic nerve. Figure 7.19A: the probe is placed temporally with its marker near the limbus. The patient directs the gaze away from the probe. Figure 7.19B: a line drawing illustrating probe/beam orientation and relation to orbital structures. Figure 7.19C: the echogram. MR = medial rectus, ON = long section of the optic nerve

Figure 7.18 The 'doughnut sign' described by Byrne and Green: transverse B-scan of a distended nerve. The outer dark outline of the distended sheaths surrounds an inner whiter circle, representing the nerve proper. This is seen when the subarachnoid space is markedly distended, as in cases of pseudotumour cerebri

of the echogram. The sections that will most easily display the nerve are L-3 in the right eye and L-9 in the left, as the probe is placed on the more accessible temporal aspect of the globe. Longitudinal sections provide additional documentation and may be the method of choice in displaying optic disc drüsen (Figure 7.20) and large cupping (Figure 7.21). By

avoidance of the lens, better imaging of the anterior third of the nerve is also obtained.

LACRIMAL GLAND EXAMINATION

Echographic examination of the lacrimal gland, particularly with A-scan, provides useful information on the nature of its lesions and their precise location and extent into the orbit.[14,15] It is worth remembering that 'non-gland' masses may occupy the lacrimal fossa region and that bilateral gland disorders are not uncommon.

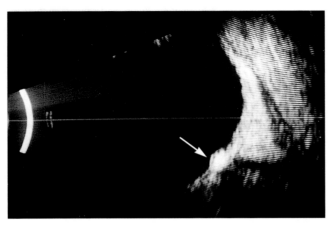

Figure 7.20 Optic disc drüsen: longitudinal B-scan section displaying a large, highly reflective nerve head (arrow) with shadowing, characteristic of optic disc drüsen

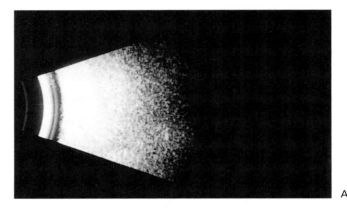

A

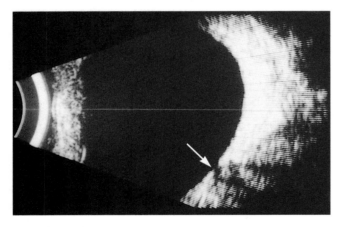

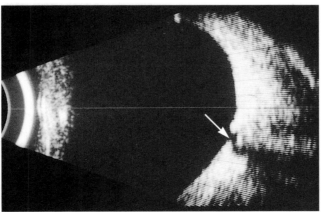

Figure 7.21 Bilateral optic disc cupping (arrows) clearly seen on longitudinal B-scan sections

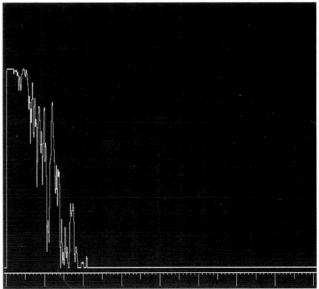

B

Figure 7.22 A- and B-scans of normal lacrimal gland (paraocular approach). The gland is indistinguishable from the surrounding orbital fat

A-scan screening

The gland is screened via the paraocular approach. The probe is firmly placed on the skin after the application of coupling jelly, and the beam is directed at the gland area, avoiding the eye pattern. A small chain of high-reflective echoes is produced, as the normal gland is too small and is indistinguishable from the surrounding fat (Figure 7.22). Abnormal lacrimal gland mass produces either widening or a defect (or both) in the fat pattern. Useful information is obtained from the reflectivity, homogeneity, and sound attenuation of the lesion spikes. Two examples are illustrated in Figures 7.23 and 7.24.

Paraocular screening of the whole of the supratemporal anterior orbit is performed and compared to that of the other orbit to detect bilateral disease. This is common in lymphoma, sarcoidosis, and viral adenitis.[16] Transocular screening of the superior and temporal orbit is helpful in detecting large lacrimal gland masses invading the deeper orbit.

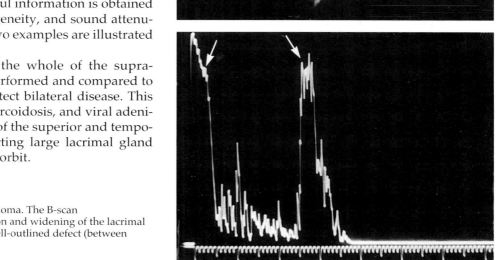

Figure 7.23 Lacrimal gland lymphoma. The B-scan shows a dark, tongue-like infiltration and widening of the lacrimal gland area. The A-scan reveals a well-outlined defect (between arrows) and a low-reflective lesion

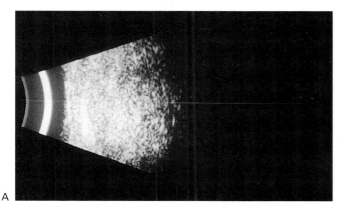

A

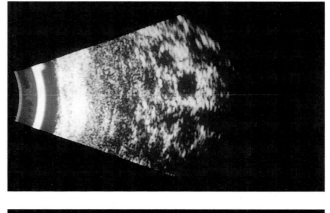

B

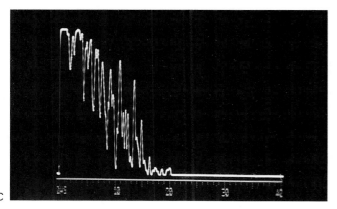

C

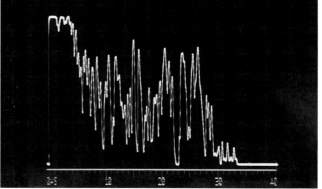

D

Figure 7.24 Acute dacryoadenitis. Figures 7.24A and 7.24C: B- and A-scans of the (normal) fellow gland. Figure 7.24B: B-scan of the involved gland, which is enlarged and contains multiple, oval, and round dark pockets, giving it a honeycomb appearance.
Figure 7.24D: A-scan of the involved gland. The pattern is widened and spikes are more heterogeneous, but the overall reflectivity remains similar to that of the normal gland

B-scan screening

The probe is placed directly on the skin, over the lacrimal gland region, after the application of coupling jelly (Figure 7.25). Transverse (marker nasally) and longitudinal (marker up) sections are obtained and compared to the contralateral orbit. Normally a homogeneous, bright echo-pattern is displayed (Figure 7.22).

An abnormal lacrimal gland lesion produces a dark outline (Figures 7.23, 7.24). Transocular B-scan will detect masses invading the deeper orbit beyond the equatorial plane of the globe; if large enough these masses may also indent the adjacent globe wall (Figure 7.26).

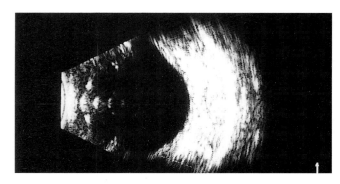

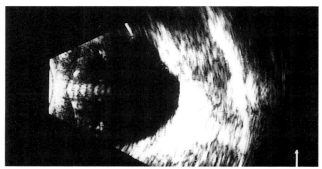

Figure 7.26 Transocular B-scan of a large lacrimal gland lesion. Figure 7.26A: the normal side. Figure 7.26B: a large dark lesion is seen in the upper orbital portion of the echogram. The adjacent globe wall is indented by the lesion

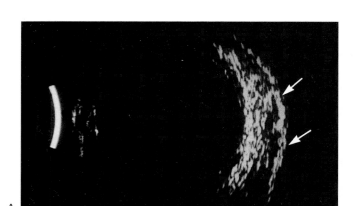

Figure 7.25 B-scan probe position for paraocular screening of a lacrimal gland

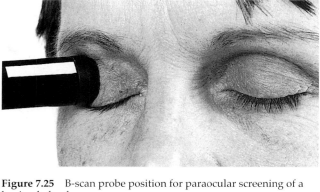

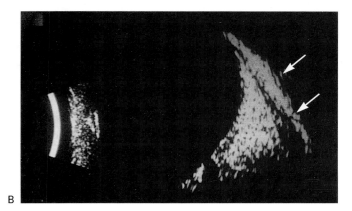

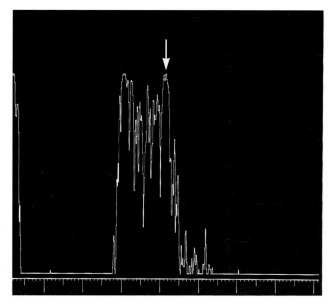

Figure 7.27 High-contrast transverse and longitudinal B-scans (Figures 7.27A and 7.27B) demonstrating orbital bone line (arrows). On A-scan (Figure 7.27C) this appears as a thick tall spike (arrow), limiting the posterior aspect of orbital fat echoes. A short chain of reverberation signals is seen beyond the bone spike

BONY WALLS AND PERIORBITA

Some orbital lesions are associated with bony defects and erosion, and an abnormal signal from the adjacent sinuses. If such lesions are suspected, radiological and MRI scanning are usually indicated to demonstrate the full extent of the bony involvement and sinus disease. Ultrasonography in these cases serves as a screening modality and may in some cases supply additional information.

Orbital bone scanning

The orbital bony wall is seen as a continuous high-reflective line on B-scan and a thick tall spike on A-scan, limiting the posterior aspect of the orbital fat echoes (Figure 7.27). The bone line is best seen on equatorial sections where the sound beam is perpendicular to the orbital wall. Sound energy is completely blocked at the bony interface, resulting in a total shadowing effect. However, reverberation signals (artefacts) are invariably seen beyond the bone echoes (Figure 7.28) and should not be confused with abnormal signals.

Malignant orbital tumours, particularly those originating from the nasopharynx, as well as mucoceles and large fractures, are common causes of erosion or interruption of the bony line (Figure 7.29). An abnormal but intact bony line may also be associated with large, slowly growing masses such as dermoid cysts and osteomas (Figure 7.30).

Examination of sinuses and lacrimal sac

The frontal, maxillary, and ethmoid sinuses are superficial enough to permit ultrasound examination. The sinuses are examined by A- and B-scan with the probe positioned directly over the corresponding area. Normally a short chain of spikes on A-scan and a narrow band of bright echoes on B-scan are obtained, as the sound propagation is interrupted by the bony wall and is no longer transmitted through air. Bony defects and fluid in the sinuses allow further propagation of sound into the sinus cavity (Figure 7.31). This is seen in cases of orbital mucoceles connected to the sinus (Figure 7.29) and in large blow-out fractures.

Direct scanning of the lacrimal sac can be performed and may be helpful in demonstrating a dacryolith (stone), which is occasionally seen in long-standing cases of lacrimal sac mucocele (Figure 7.32).

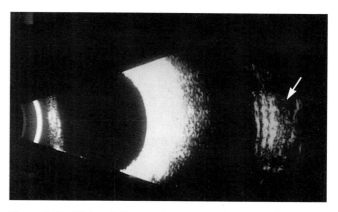

Figure 7.28 High-gain B-scan showing reverberation echoes behind the orbit (arrow). These are located at a distance of 'one eye-length' from the posterior globe wall

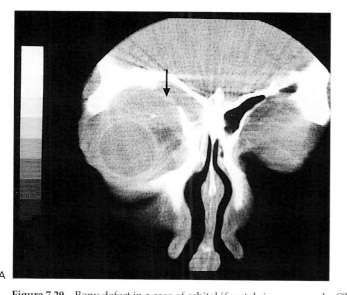

A

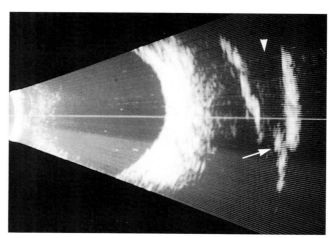

B

Figure 7.29 Bony defect in a case of orbital/frontal sinus mucocele: CT scan (Figure 7.29A) showing a bone defect and communication to an opaque frontal sinus (arrow). The B-scan (Figure 7.29B) demonstrates a diffuse low-reflective orbital lesion, and an interruption of the bone line (arrow). An abnormal sinus signal is also present (arrow head)

113

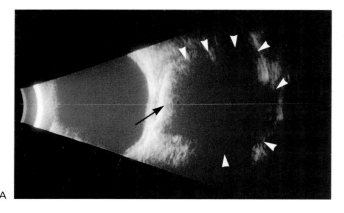

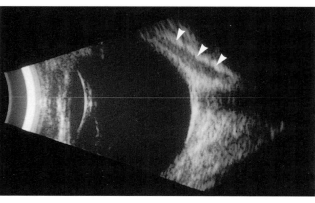

A

C

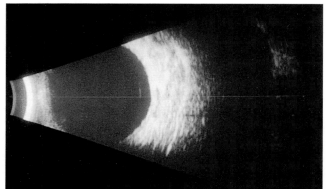

B

Figure 7.30 Orbital osteoma. Figure 7.30A: a transverse B-scan of the nasal orbital cavity. A large, round, very low reflective lesion is seen occupying most of the orbital space (arrow heads). The bone line is pressed forward against an indented globe wall (long arrow). Figure 7.30B: the same region in the fellow orbit. Figure 7.30C: a horizontal axial scan presenting another view of the abnormal bone line nasally (arrow heads)

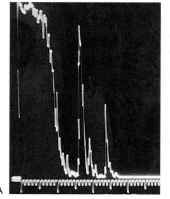

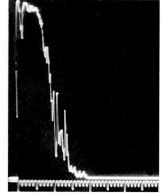

A

B

Figure 7.31 Abnormal sinus signal. Figure 7.31A is an A-scan of an abnormal frontal sinus, showing a more highly reflective and wider pattern than that of the normal sinus (Figure 7.31B).

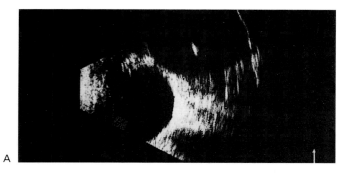

A

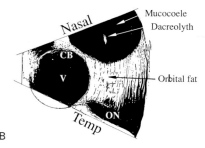

B

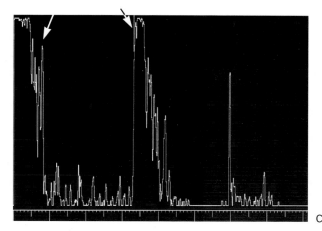

C

Figure 7.32 B-scan (Figure 7.32A) and line drawing (Figure 7.32B) of a large, low-reflective, lacrimal sac mucocele. A high-reflective echo-source, representing a dacryolith, is also seen (CB = ciliary body, V = vitreous cavity). Figure 7.32C is the A-scan. The mucocele is well outlined (arrows). A low-reflective chain of spikes within the lesion indicates a thick, purulent consistency of the sac contents

DOPPLER ULTRASOUND

Great advances have recently been made in the development of Doppler ultrasound. New features include combined Doppler and B-scan (Duplex scanning), colour flow mapping, and facilities for measuring flow direction and blood velocity. The result is a more impressive display of lesions and accurate quantification of blood flow characteristics.

The Doppler principle,[17] vividly illustrated by the frequency shift of the siren of a moving police car, is presented in the following equation:

$$Fd = Ft - Fr = 2 \, V \, Ft \cos 0 / c$$

where Fd is the difference in frequency (Doppler shift), Ft the transmitted frequency, Fr the received frequency, V the velocity of blood flow, 0 the angle of incidence of the sound beam on the blood vessel, and c the velocity of ultrasound in tissue. From the above equation, it can be shown that a stronger Doppler signal is obtained if the velocity of blood flow is increased and, more importantly for the examiner, if the ultrasound beam is directed at a more acute angle to the blood vessel (Figure 7.33). A compromise therefore exists, in duplex scanners, between perpendicular B-scan beam and angled Doppler beam for the purpose of obtaining an optimum signal. This is taken into account in the design of duplex probes, where a 90° placement of the B-probe coincides with a 30–60° orientation of the Doppler probe.

In practice, Doppler ultrasound is employed for flow detection using non-directional continuous wave

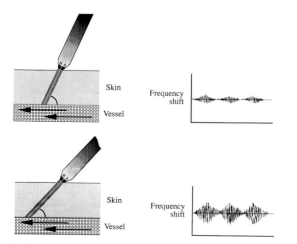

Figure 7.33 Effect of the angle of the incident ultrasound beam on the Doppler frequency shift. A higher frequency is obtained, with a more acute angle. No signal is obtained if the probe is oriented at right angles to the blood vessel, (A = transmitting crystal; B = receiving crystal)

(CW) Doppler, and for volumetric flow and velocity quantification and wave-form analysis, using pulsed-wave (PW) Doppler. Recently, PW Doppler has been incorporated, as an additional imaging technique, in Duplex scanners and in colour flow mapping.

Continuous-wave (CW) Doppler

This is the simplest mode. A crystal continuously transmits and another continuously receives echoes. CW Doppler, with a signal frequency of 5–10 MHz is used in the orbit for flow detection, and supplies qualitative data on the vascularity of lesions and on abnormal or asymmetrical increases in orbital blood flow.[18] CW Doppler, however, has no depth resolution and therefore does not supply information on blood velocity or flow volume measurements.

Technique of examination with CW Doppler

The probe may be placed directly on the globe or on the closed eyelids after the application of coupling jelly (Figure 7.34). Doppler examination is best carried out after localization of lesions with A- and B-scans. An arterial (pulsatile), venous (continuous), or mixed signal may be obtained. The signal is maximized by fine adjustments of the probe position and it is then compared with the same position in the other orbit.

Normally an audible signal is obtained over the lacrimal gland area, the supra-nasal orbit, and the optic nerve. The echographer is advised to examine many normal orbits in order to become familiar with the technique and to be able to differentiate between normal and abnormal signals.

Examples of orbital lesions producing an abnormal Doppler signal include carotid-cavernous and dural sinus fistulae, capillary haemangioma, and optic nerve meningiomas. An increase in the 'normal' Doppler signal may occasionally be encountered when a normal vascular tissue is pushed nearer to the surface by a deeper 'Doppler silent' mass. It is helpful in these cases to obtain occurate A- and B-scans before Doppler assessment is carried out.

Duplex scanning and colour flow imaging

The application of these techniques is relatively new in ophthalmology.[19,20,21,22] The appeal of simultaneously transmitting B-scan images with Doppler signals is obvious (Figure 7.35). In colour flow mapping, the grey-scale B-scan is combined with a colour-coded signal determined by the Doppler shift, where different shades of red and blue represent arterial and venous flow at different velocities. In Duplex scanning the velocity of blood can also be determined by measuring the angle between the Doppler beam and blood vessel.

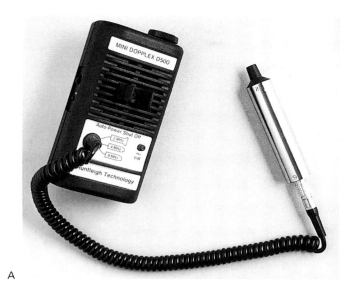

A

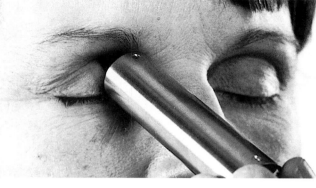

B

Figure 7.34 (A) An example of a hand-held continuous-wave Doppler for ophthalmic use. A choice of 2, 4, and 8 MHz probes is available. (B) The probe is placed firmly on the area of interest, after applying coupling jelly on the skin

Both techniques, however, are still subject to the physical laws governing Doppler ultrasound and the compromise, described above, between the optimum (perpendicular) angle of B-scan image and the acute angle of Doppler ultrasound.

Duplex scanners and colour flow mapping are now being used to examine vascularity in ocular melanomas[21,23,24] and orbital lesions[24,25] and to detect normal and abnormal blood flow in the ophthalmic and central retinal vessels[25,26,27] and in ischaemic optic neuropathy.[28]

Figure 7.35 Duplex scanning of the orbit. The sample area for Doppler – in this case that of the optic nerve (central retinal artery) – can be selected on B-scan (arrow). The Doppler frequency shift is simultaneously displayed

REFERENCES

1 Byrne S F, Glaser J S. Orbital tissue differentiation with standardized echography. Ophthalomology 1983; 90:1071–1090
2 Byrne S F, Green R L. Orbital echography. In: Tasman W, Jaeger E A (eds) Duane's clinical ophthalmology, Vol 2, Ch 26. Philadelphia: Lippincott, 1991
3 Dick A D, Nangia V, Atta H R. Standardised echography in the differential diagnosis of extraocular muscle enlargement. Eye 1992; 6:610–617
4 Byrne S F, Gendron E K, Glaser J S et al. Diameter of normal extraocular recti muscles with echography. Am J Ophthalmol 1991; 112:706–713
5 Byrne S F. Evaluation of the optic nerve with standardized echography. In: Smith J L (ed) Neuro ophthalmology now. New York: Field, Raicha, 1986:45–66
6 Atta H R. Imaging of the optic nerve with standardized echography. Eye 1988; 2:358–366
7 Ossoinig K C. Standardized echography of the optic nerve, Jules Francois Memorial Lecture. In: Till P (ed) Ophthalmic Echography 13. Dordrecht: Kluwer, 1993:3–99
8 Ossoinig K C, Cennamo G, Byrne S F. Echographic differential diagnosis of optic nerve lesions. Doc Ophthalmol Pro Ser 1981; 29:327–331
9 Lawton Smith J, Hoyt W F, Newton T H. Optic nerve sheath decompression for relief of chronic monocular choked disc. Am J Ophthalmol 1969; 68:633–639
10 Conn H, Tenzel R R, Lawton Smith J. Optic disc changes with intracranial subarachnoid cysts. J Clin Neuro-Ophthalmol 1982; 2:183–192
11 Hupp S L, Glaser J S, Byrne S F. Optic nerve sheath decompression. Arch Ophthalmol 1987; 105:386–389
12 Hamed L M, Tse D T, Glaser J S et al. Neuroimaging of the optic nerve after fenestration for management of pseudotumour cerebri. Arch Ophthalmol 1992; 110:636–639
13 Hasenfratz G. Experimental studies on the display of the optic nerve. In: Ossoinig K C (ed) Ophthalmic echography. Dordrecht: Junk, 1987:587–602

14 Byrne S F, Green R L. Ultrasound of the eye and orbit. St Louis: Mosby Year Book, 1992:405–407

15 Balchunas W R, Quencer R M, Byrne S F. Lacrimal gland and fossa masses: evaluation by computed tomography and A-mode echography. Radiology 1983; 149:751–758

16 Rootman J, Lapointe J S. Tumours of the lacrimal gland. In: Rootman J (ed) Diseases of the orbit. Philadelphia: Lippincott, 1988:386

17 Atkinson P, Woodcock J P. Doppler ultrasound and its use in clinical measurement. Medical Physics Series, Academic Press, London 1982

18 Nisbet R M, Barber J C, Steinkuller P G. Doppler ultrasonic flow detector: an adjunct in evaluation of orbital lesions. J Pediatr Ophthalmol Strabismus 1980; 17:268

19 Erickson S J, Hendrix L E, Massaro B M et al. Color Doppler flow imaging of the normal and abnormal orbit. Radiology 1989; 173:511–516

20 Lieb W E, Cohen S M, Merton D A et al. Color Doppler imaging of the eye and orbit. Technique and normal vascular anatomy. Arch Ophthalmol 1991; 109:527–531

21 Guthoff R, Berger R W, Helmke K et al. Doppler sonographische Befunde bei intraokularen Tumoren. Fortschr Ophthalmol 1989; 86:239–241

22 Flaharty P M, Lieb W E, Sergott R C et al. Color Doppler imaging. A new non-invasive technique to diagnose and monitor carotid-cavernous sinus fistula. Arch Ophthalmol 1991; 109: 522–526

23 Guthoff R, Berger R W, Winkler P et al. Doppler ultrasonography of malignant melanomas of the uvea. Arch Ophthalmol 1991; 109:537–541

24 Lieb W E, Flaharty P M, Ho A et al. Color Doppler imaging of the eye and orbit. A synopsis of a 400 case experience. Acta Ophthalmologica (Suppl. 204) 1992; 70:50–54

25 Aburn N S, Sergott R C. Orbital colour Doppler imaging. Eye 1993; 7:639–647

26 Guthoff R, Berger R W, Winkler P et al. Doppler ultrasonography of the ophthalmic and central retinal vessels. Arch Ophthalmol 1991; 109:532–536

27 Williamson T H, Baxter G M, Dutton G N. Colour Doppler velocimetry of the arterial vasculature of the optic nerve head and orbit. Eye 1993; 7:74–79

28 Williamson T H, Baxter G, Paul R et al. Colour Doppler ultrasound in the management of a case of cranial arteritis. Br J Ophthalmol 1992; 76:690–691

8

Special examination techniques: orbit

In this section the 'special techniques' described in Chapter 4 for the eye will be applied to the echographic diagnosis of orbital diseases (Table 7.1). In addition to quantitative, kinetic, and topographic echography, Doppler ultrasound is utilized as part of the kinetic examination to evaluate orbital blood flow and the vascularity of its lesions.

As in the ocular section, these techniques will be demonstrated in relation to some of the commonly encountered orbital disorders, namely enlargement of the extraocular muscles, vascular lesions, and orbital masses.

Table 8.1 Causes of enlarged extraocular muscles	
Cause	No. (%)
Thyroid orbitopathy	64 (81.0)
Orbital myositis	5 (6.3)
Orbital venous congestion	4 (5.0)
Metastatic disease	4 (5.0)
Lymphoma	1 (1.3)
Lithium therapy	1 (1.3)
Total	79 (100)

ENLARGEMENT OF THE EXTRAOCULAR MUSCLES

The most common cause of enlargement of extraocular muscles is thyroid orbitopathy. This is followed by orbital myositis, orbital venous congestion, neoplasm, granuloma, muscle haematoma, and lithium therapy.[1,2] Table 8.1 summarizes an incidence of enlarged extraocular muscles, as diagnosed on echography in a period of one year.

Thyroid orbitopathy

In the *topographic* evaluation, swelling is maximally seen at the belly and more posteriorly, while the insertion is relatively spared (Figure 8.1). More than one muscle is normally enlarged and both orbits are invariably affected, even in the absence of clinical signs.[3,4] Muscle measurements tend to vary during the course of the disease. Other findings include widening of orbital fat and thickening of periosteum (space between muscle and bony wall) (Figure 8.2), enlargement of the lacrimal gland, and, in severe cases, distension of the optic nerve and engorgement of orbital veins;[5] this is best seen in the supra-nasal orbital space (Figure 8.3). If optic nerve compression is suspected, further investigations and orbital decompression must be considered.

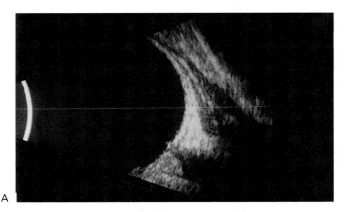

A

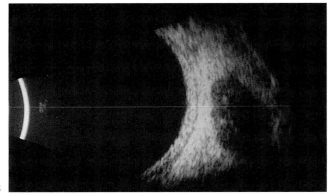

B

Figure 8.1 Thyroid orbitopathy. Longitudinal (Figure 8.1A) and transverse (Figure 8.1B) B-scans showing marked swelling of a medial rectus muscle. Swelling is maximally seen at the belly, with the insertion relatively spared

Quantitative echography assesses the reflectivity of the muscle. Normally, the rectus muscles exhibit medium to medium/high spikes on A-scan (Figure 7.8). In early orbitopathy the reflectivity may not be altered or may be slightly reduced, probably as a result of oedema and cellular infiltration between muscle fibres (Figure 8.4). In long-standing cases an increase in the spikes' height is observed, presumably because of fibrosis (Figure 8.5); this occasionally makes it difficult to isolate the characteristic muscle defect from the surrounding fat.

Kinetic echography entails examination of the optic nerve and performance of the 30° test (p. 106) to detect optic nerve compression. This is a good positive test in thyroid orbitopathy. A negative 30° test, however, does not exclude 'chronic' compression of the optic nerve. In such cases the diagnosis is reached clinically and by other 'optic nerve investigations'. Kinetic examination, including Doppler ultrasound, is also helpful in detecting enlarged orbital veins and increased venous phase on Doppler. This is seen in severe compressive orbitopathy that produces obstruction of the orbital venous outflow.

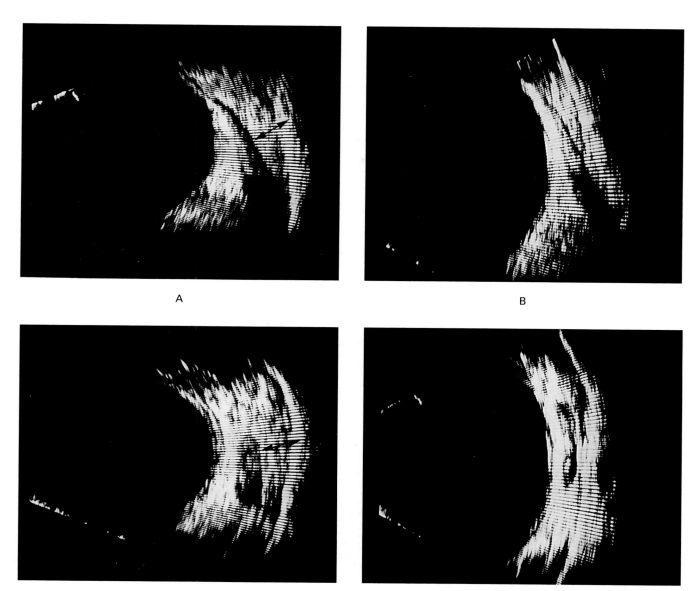

A

B

Figure 8.2 Thyroid orbitopathy. Scans of an affected orbit (Figure 8.2A) compared to those of the contralateral 'normal' orbit (Figure 8.2B). In addition to muscle enlargement, there is a general increase (widening) of the fat segment and thickening of periosteum (i.e. space between muscle and bone line) (double-ended arrow)

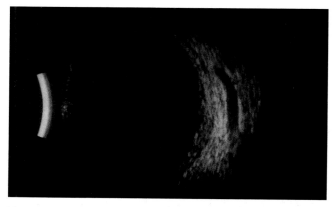

Figure 8.3 Engorgement of an orbital vein encountered in severe, compressive thyroid orbitopathy. This appears as a dark tubular structure, usually seen at the supra-nasal orbital space

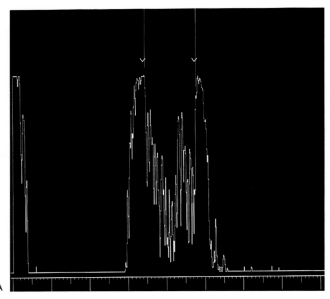

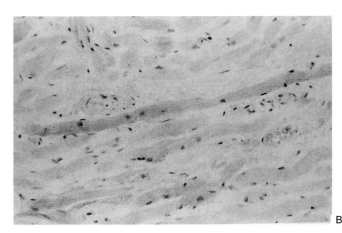

Figure 8.4 Early thyroid myopathy. Figure 8.4A: A-scan showing a markedly enlarged muscle (between arrows) early in the course of the disease. The overall reflectivity of the muscle is lower than normal. Figure 8.4B: histological section showing oedema and cellular infiltrate between muscle fibres

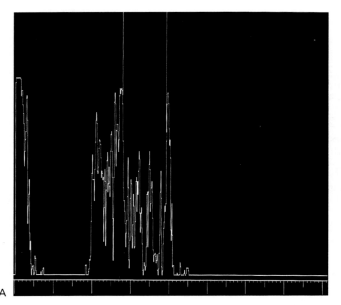

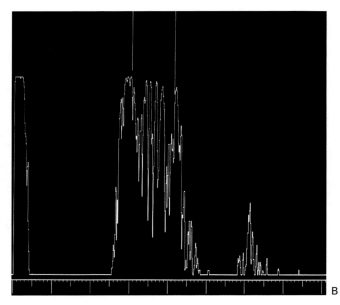

Figure 8.5 Late thyroid myopathy. Figure 8.5A: an A-scan of an enlarged medial rectus muscle soon after diagnosis. Figure 8.5B: A-scan of the same muscle many months later. Note the marked increase in reflectivity of the muscle fibres

Orbital myositis

On *topographic* examination only one muscle is usually affected. All extraocular muscles, however, are susceptible, including the obliques.[6] Thickening involves the insertion as well as the belly (Figure 8.6).[1,5] Other findings may include adjacent posterior scleritis – with or without extension along the optic nerve sheaths – giving rise to the characteristic 'T-sign' (Figure 8.7) and an inflammatory 'pseudotumour' mass in the surrounding fat.[7,8]

On *quantitative* examination the reflectivity of the muscle is greatly reduced (Figure 8.8).[1,5,6] Both reflectivity and muscle diameter return to normal following the introduction of systemic steroid therapy. The therapeutic effect of steroids can therefore be monitored on echography as well as clinically, helping to prevent a recurrence due to early withdrawal of treatment.

Kinetic and *Doppler* echography do not yield positive findings in cases of orbital myositis. A normal Doppler response, however, will rule out orbital venous congestion as a cause.

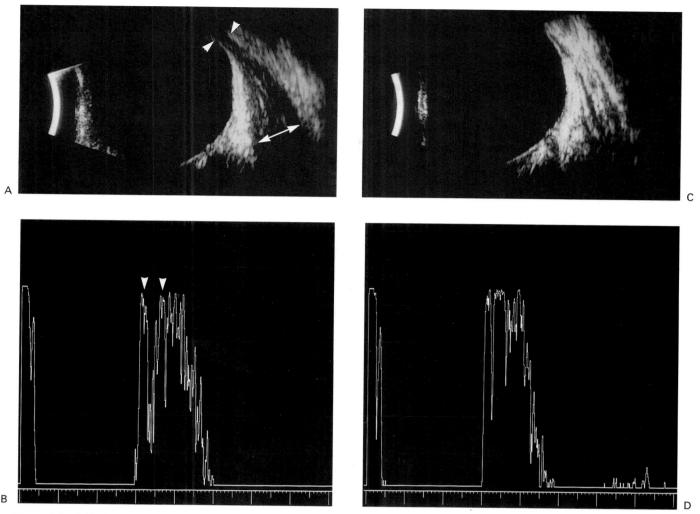

Figure 8.6 Orbital myositis. Figure 8.6A: a longitudinal B-scan of an affected medial rectus. Figure 8.6B: an A-scan of its insertion. The insertion is thickened, as seen on B- and A-scans (arrow heads). The belly is markedly distended on B-scan (double-ended arrow). Figures 8.6C and 8.6D are the same scans of the opposite, normal medial rectus

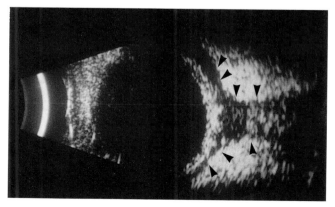

Figure 8.7 Orbital myositis associated with posterior scleritis. A low-reflective thickened episcleral space extends along the optic nerve sheaths, giving rise to the 'T-sign' (arrow heads)

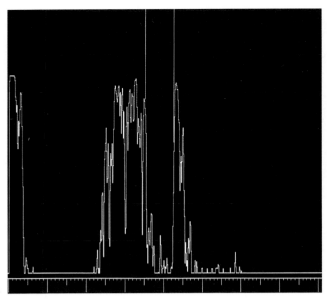
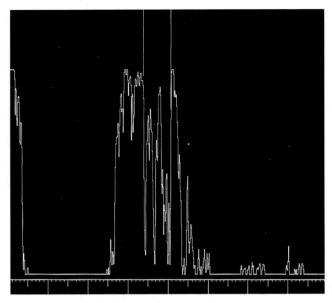

Figure 8.8 Orbital myositis: quantitative assessment. Figure 8.8A: A-scan of an affected muscle, showing greatly reduced reflectivity. Figure 8.8B: the same muscle following systemic corticosteroid therapy. Note the significant increase in muscle reflectivity, which is returning to the normal level

Table 8.2 Echographic differentiation of extraocular muscle swelling			
Technique	Thyroid orbitopathy	Myositis	Orbital venous congestion
Topographic	Variable muscles Bilateral Insertion spared	Single muscle Unilateral Insertion thickened	All muscles Uni/bilateral Insertion spared
Quantitative	Normal reflectivity or increased (late)	Reduced	Normal reflectivity
Other findings	Thickened optic nerve Widening of fat Normal Doppler	Posterior scleritis Normal Doppler	Enlarged orbital vein Distended optic nerve Abnormal Doppler

Table 8.2 summarizes the echographic differentiation of extraocular muscle enlargement.

VASCULAR LESIONS IN THE ORBIT

Vascular lesions constitute one of the most frequent causes of orbital disease.[9,10] Three such lesions are discussed: arterio-venous fistula, orbital varices, and capillary haemangioma.

Arterio-venous fistula

A high flow, carotid-cavernous fistula produces an acute and severe engorgement of the orbital venous system, while a dural sinus (low-flow) fistula is more insidious, resulting in less spectacular orbital signs.[11] The main echographic finding is an enlarged orbital vein, particularly the superior ophthalmic, which can easily be seen on B-scan.[12] This appears as a dark 'sausage-like' outline in the supra-nasal aspect of the orbit (Figure 8.9). Cross- and longitudinal sections of the vein can be obtained (Figure 8.10).

Other *topographic* findings include a uniform enlargement of all the extraocular muscles (from venous engorgement) and, in severe cases, distension of the optic nerve sheaths, disc oedema (Figure 8.9), and thickening or detachment of the chorio-retinal layer.

Quantitative A-scan examination identifies and measures the thickness of the enlarged vein, muscles, and optic nerve.

Kinetic and *Doppler* echography are very helpful in demonstrating vascularity in the enlarged vein.[11,13,14]

On A-scan, this appears as fast vertical vibrations of spikes within the vessel. Vascularity can be very pronounced in carotid-cavernous fistula but mild in dural–sinus fistula. The Doppler signal is arterialized and loud. The vein can be made to collapse on B-scan by applying firm pressure on the globe with the probe (Figure 8.10). Distension of the nerve sheaths is also assessed dynamically using the 30° test, but this may be difficult to elicit because of proptosis and restriction of eye movements.

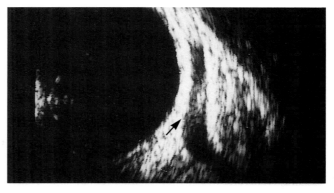

A

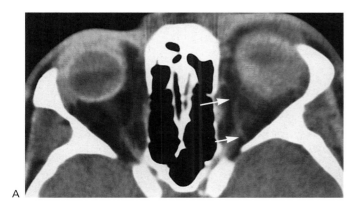

A

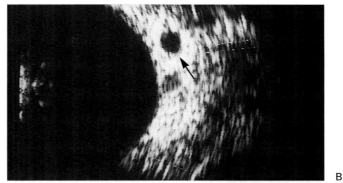

B

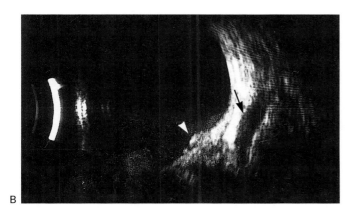

B

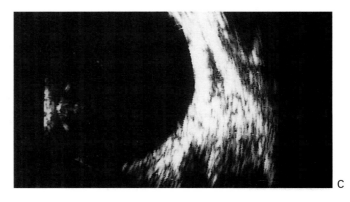

C

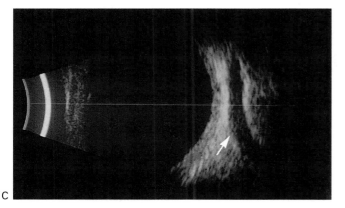

C

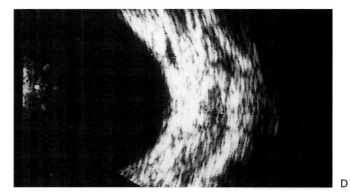

D

Figure 8.9 Enlarged orbital vein. Figure 8.9A: CT scan showing the normal anatomical course of the superior ophthalmic vein, winding its way over the optic nerve from the antero-nasal to the postero-temporal region (arrows). Figures 8.9B and 8.9C: examples of enlarged orbital veins (arrows) detected in the supra-nasal orbital space. Disc oedema is also seen in the middle echogram (arrow head)

Figure 8.10 Kinetic evaluation of an enlarged orbital vein. Figures 8.10A and 8.10B: long and cross-sections of an enlarged orbital vein (arrows) before the application of pressure on the globe. Figures 8.10C and 8.10D: the same scans after the application of pressure, showing collapse of the vein

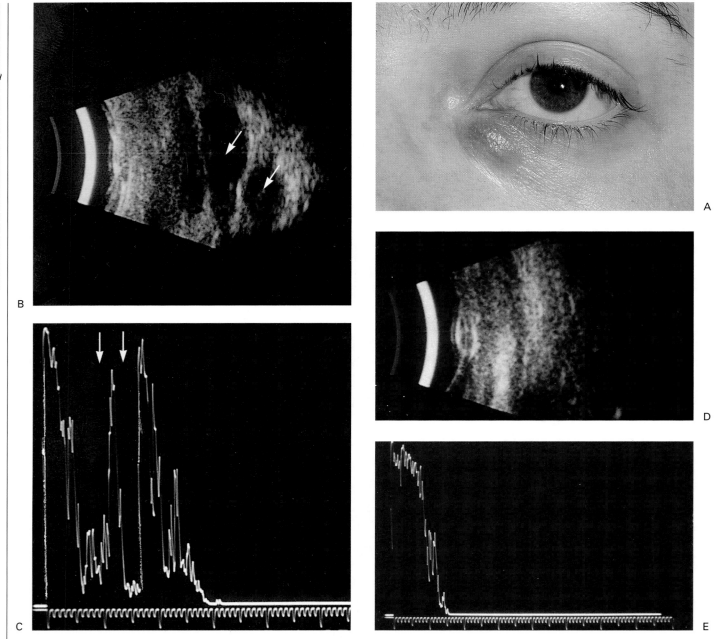

Figure 8.11 Orbital varix. Figure 8.11A: clinical photograph showing a blue-grey, soft, subcutaneous lesion in the lower lid. Paraocular B- and A-scans (Figures 8.11B and 8.11C) revealed multiple low-reflective channels (arrows), best seen during Valsalva's manoeuvre. The channels appear to collapse after Valsalva (Figures 8.11D and 8.11E)

Orbital varices (venous malformation)

These lesions are a frequent cause of intermittent proptosis in the first two decades of life.[9,15] The classic *topographic* feature is that of a low-reflective, tubular, vein-like, or irregular channel, usually located anteriorly and nasally in the orbit.[16] Many lesions are located so anteriorly that they may only be seen on paraocular examination.

Kinetic examination shows the lesion 'opening up' or expanding during Valsalva manoeuvre and collapsing after stopping Valsalva or upon compression of the globe.[15,16] Unlike A-V fistula, no other congestive orbital signs are seen and vascularity within the enlarged vein is minimal or absent. Figures 8.11 and 8.12 illustrate two examples of orbital varices.

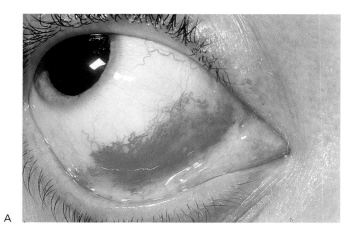

A

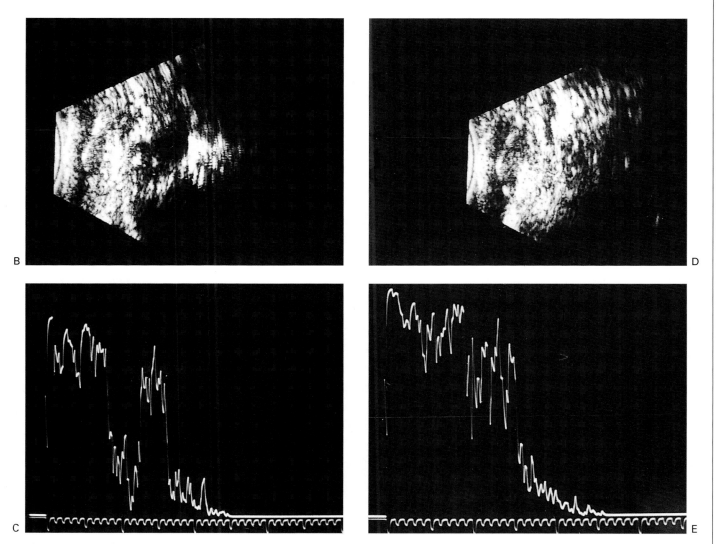

Figure 8.12 Another example of an orbital varix. Clinically, the lesion is located under the conjunctiva (Figure 8.12A). B- and A-scans during Valsalva (Figures 8.12B and 8.12C) show a large, single, low-reflective channel, which disappears after Valsalva (Figures 8.12D and 8.12E)

Capillary haemangioma

This lesion commonly presents at birth or in early life.[9,10] In superficially placed lesions the diagnosis is easily reached clinically by observation of the characteristic 'port-wine' skin stain. The detection of deeper lesions in the orbit can be aided by echography.[16]

Topographically, capillary haemangioma appears as either a poorly or a well outlined lesion, located deep inside or outside the muscle cone, or preseptally where it is best demonstrated on paraocular sections.

On *quantitative* assessment, the heterogeneous histological character of capillary haemangioma gives rise to an irregular internal structure with alternate high and low reflectivity.

Capillary haemangioma is a vascular lesion.[7] On *kinetic* examination, fine vertical oscillations of tumour spikes are observed on A-scan. An increased signal on Doppler ultrasound may also be noted. Vascularity, however, can be variable and is difficult to detect in some cases. On exertion of pressure with the B-scan probe, capillary haemangioma also tends to compress. Figure 8.13 illustrates the echographic appearance of a capillary haemangioma in a 9-month-old girl.

Table 8.3 summarizes the echographic features of the three vascular lesions.

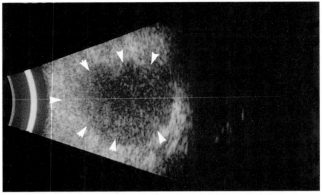

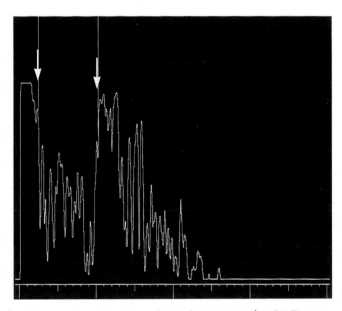

Figure 8.13 Capillary haemangioma. Figure 8.13A: paraocular B-scan showing a poorly outlined round mass lesion (arrow heads). Figures 8.13B and 8.13C: paraocular A-scans of the lesion taken at different angles, and illustrating the heterogeneity of its internal structure (between arrows)

Table 8.3	Echographic features of common orbital vascular lesions		
Technique	A-V fistula	Orbital varix	Capillary haemangioma
Topographic	Tubular outline Sharp borders Supra-nasal, deep orbit	Tortuous outline Sharp borders Antero-nasal, superficial	Mass lesion Variable Variable
Quantitative	Low-reflective Regular internal structure Weak sound attenuation	Low-reflective Regular internal structure Weak sound attenuation	Variable/high Irregular Irregular
Kinetic	Pronounced vascularity Collapses on moderate pressure Mobile Valsalva inconclusive (dangerous)	Absent/minimal Collapses on minimal pressure Mobile Valsalva highly positive	Absent/minimal Variable, soft to firm Immobile Valsalva negative

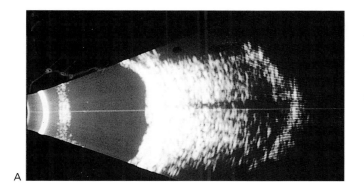

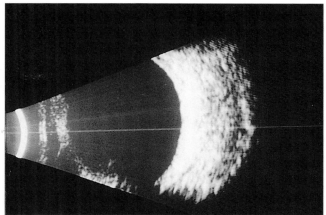

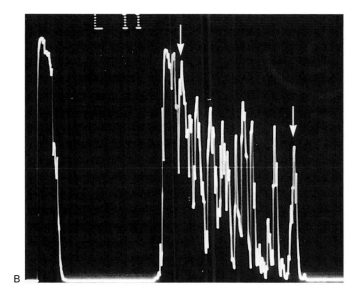

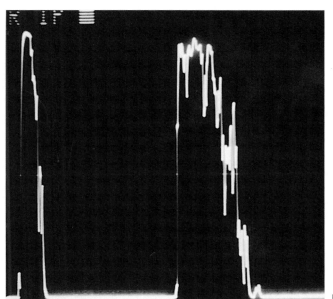

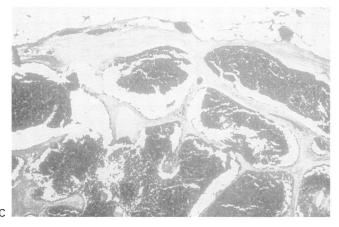

A

D

B

E

C

Figure 8.14 Cavernous haemangioma. Figure 8.14A: B-scan showing a large, round mass, occupying almost the entire orbital space and indenting the globe. Figure 8.14B: the lesion (between arrows) is moderately high reflective and shows significant sound attenuation. The spikes' pattern is regular, consisting of high-alternating with low-reflective echoes, which are characteristic of this lesion and reflect the honeycombed, vacuolar histological structure (Figure 8.14C). Figures 8.14D and 8.14E: the normal fellow orbit

ORBITAL MASS LESION

Three examples of orbital mass lesions are described: cavernous haemangioma, pseudotumour/lymphoma, and orbital mucocele.

Cavernous haemangioma

This lesion is one of the most common primary orbital tumours in adults.[17,18] The classical clinical presentation is that of a slow, progressive, and painless proptosis with no significant inflammatory signs or visual disturbance, except in the late stages when a large tumour may compress the optic nerve.

Topographically, the lesion is frequently located within the muscle cone, where a large, well-outlined,

129

round or oval mass is observed. The tumour typically attains a large size before significant symptoms and signs occur. The extraocular muscles and optic nerve may be displaced around the tumour and the globe may also be indented, resulting in the common associated feature of choroidal folds.

Quantitative examination with A-scan reveals a characteristic cavernous pattern consisting of evenly spaced, alternate high- and low-reflective spikes fading gradually from left to right.[16] This is explained by the honeycomb histological structure of (highly reflective) septa and (low-reflective) blood-filled spaces evenly distributed throughout the tumour.

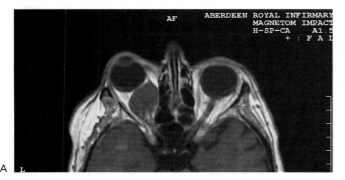

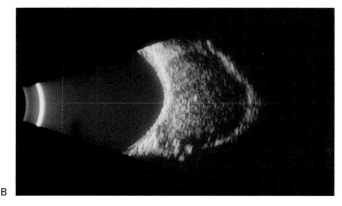

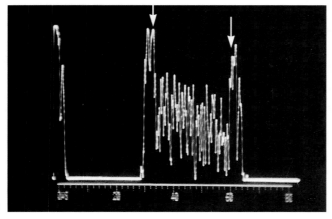

Figure 8.15 Another example of a cavernous haemangioma. Figure 8.15A: MRI scan showing an oval, nasal intra-conal mass and proptosis. Figure 8.15B: B-scan. The lesion is well outlined with a 'granular' internal structure. Figure 8.15C: A-scan demonstrating a well-outlined defect (arrows) and the typical internal structure

Kinetic echography shows a firm, poorly compressible lesion. Although a vascular tumour in origin (hamartoma), cavernous haemangioma exhibits no vascularity on A-scan or Doppler, as it is fed and drained by a small vessel(s), resulting in a very slow or stagnant blood flow or even clotting of blood within the loculi.

Figures 8.14 and 8.15 present two examples of cavernous haemangioma.

Pseudotumour/lymphoma

Although clinically different, pseudotumour and lymphoma have many common features on echography.

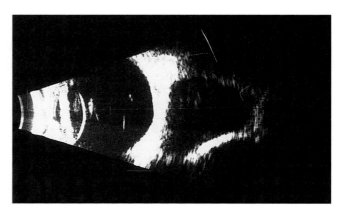

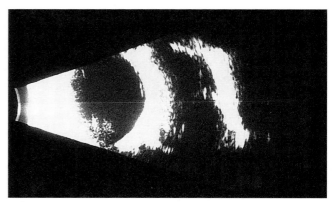

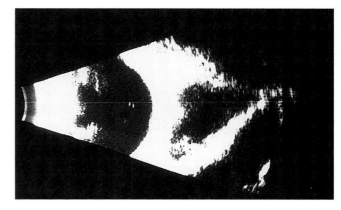

Figure 8.16 Orbital pseudotumour/lymphoma: three B-scan sections of an intra-conal pseudotumour demonstrating its irregular outline and infiltrative nature

The *topographic* appearance on B-scan consists of a poorly outlined, infiltrative, dark mass lesion with irregular borders (Figure 8.16). Both lesions can be found anywhere in the orbit, including the lacrimal gland and fossa. Unlike inflammatory pseudotumour, lymphomas may present bilaterally. Pseudotumour may be accompanied by other inflammatory signs such as orbital myositis and posterior scleritis.[8,19]

Quantitative assessment reveals very low reflectivity, regular internal structure, and weak sound attenuation (Figure 8.17). Apart from the occasional higher spikes produced by fibrous septa, the low reflectivity is attributed to the dense cellular composition of these lesions.

Kinetic examination demonstrates a firm mass with no vascularity.

Orbital mucocele

Orbital mucoceles are often connected to the frontal and ethmoid sinuses (Figure 8.18).

Topographically they are located nasally or supra-nasally in the orbit,[20] and are easily detected on paraocular examination (Figure 8.19). On B-scan,

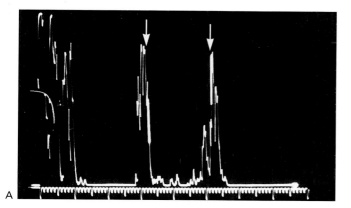
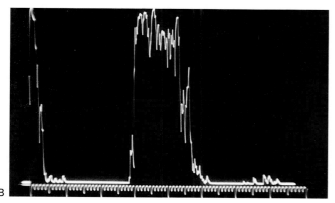

Figure 8.17 Orbital pseudotumour/lymphoma: quantitative A-scan. Figure 8.17A: the lesion (between arrows) is very low reflective with weak sound attenuation, compared to the normal orbit (Figure 8.17B)

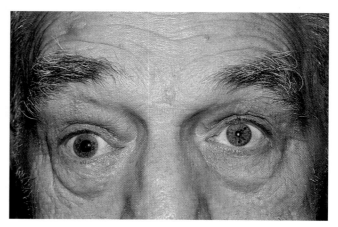

Figure 8.18 Clinical photograph of a right frontal mucocele producing proptosis and infra-temporal globe displacement

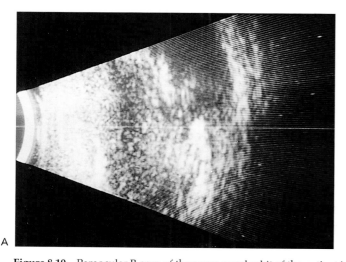
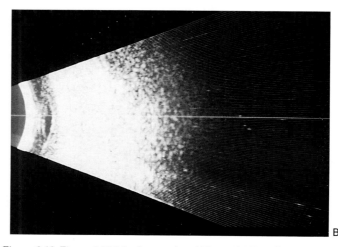

Figure 8.19 Paraocular B-scan of the supra-nasal orbit of the patient in Figure 8.18. Figure 8.19A is abnormal and Figure 8.19B is the normal side

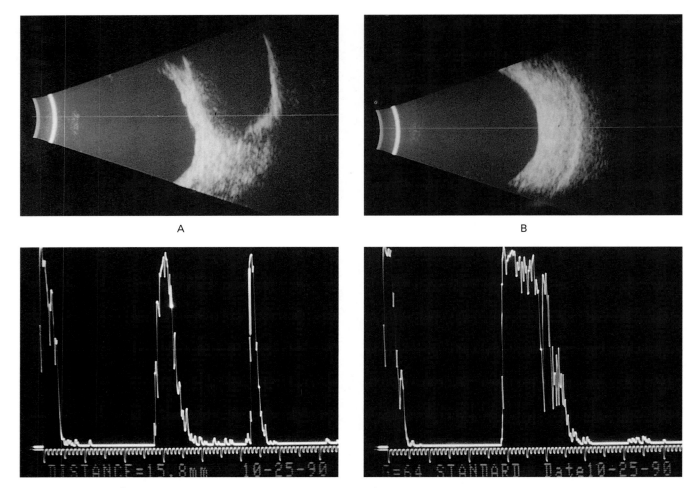

Figure 8.20 Large ethmoid mucocele. Figure 8.20A: nasal B- and A-scans showing a well-outlined, very low reflective lesion. Figure 8.20B: the normal contralateral orbit

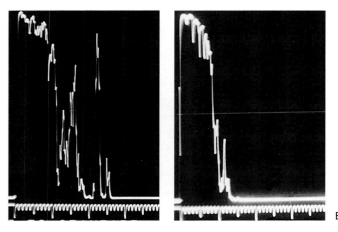

Figure 8.21 Abnormal sinus signal. Figure 8.21A: an A-scan of an abnormal frontal sinus, showing widening and irregularity of the pattern, compared to the normal sinus (Figure 8.21B)

orbital mucocele appears as a dark mass lesion (Figure 8.20). The presence of a bony defect is characteristic (Figure 7.29), as is an abnormal signal from the adjacent sinus (Figure 8.21).

Quantitative echography reveals a low or medium reflective, regularly structured lesion with weak sound attenuation (Figure 8.20).[21] An infected mucocele, however, will show an increase in reflectivity and heterogeneity.

On *kinetic* examination the lesion is firm, noncompressible, and avascular.

Table 8.4 summarizes the echographic features of these masses.

Table 8.4 Echographic differentiation of orbital mass lesion

Technique	Cavernous haemangioma	Pseudotumour/lymphoma	Mucocele
Topographic	Intra-conal Round/oval Well-outlined	Variable Irregular Poorly outlined	Supra-nasal Variable Well-outlined and bony defect
Quantitative	Medium-reflective Honeycomb structure Medium sound attenuation	Low-reflective Regular structure Low attenuation	Low/medium-reflective Regular structure Low attenuation
Kinetic	Poorly compressible Weakly vascular	Non-compressible Avascular	Non-compressible Avascular

REFERENCES

1 Dick A D, Nangia V, Atta H. Standardized echography in the differential diagnosis of extraocular muscle enlargement. Eye 6:610–617 1992

2 Ossoinig K C, Hermsen V M. Myositis of extraocular muscles diagnosed with standardized echography. In: Hillman J S, Lemay M M (eds) Ophthalmic ultrasonography. Dordrecht: Junk, 1983:381–392

3 Atta H R, McCreath G, McKillop J H et al. Ophthalmopathy in early thyrotoxicosis – relationship to thyroid receptor antibodies and effects of treatment. Scot Med J 35:41–44 1990

4 Forrester J V, Sutherland G R, McDougall I R. Dysthyroid ophthalmopathy: orbital evaluation with B-scan ultrasonography. J Clin Endocrinol and Metabolism 45:221–224 1977

5 Ossoinig K C. Ultrasonic diagnosis of Graves' ophthalmopathy. In: Gorman C A, Waller R D, Dyer J A (eds) The eye and orbit in thyroid disease. New York: Raven Press, 1984:185–211

6 Wan W L, Cano M R, Green R L. Orbital myositis involving the oblique muscles. An echographic study. Ophthalmology 95:1522–1528 1988

7 Byrne S F, Green R L. Ultrasound of the eye and orbit. St Louis: Mosby Year Book, 1992:379

8 Kennerdell J S, Dresner S C. The nonspecific orbital inflammatory syndromes. Surv Ophthalmol 29:93–103 1984

9 Wright J E. Current concepts in orbital disease. Doyne Lecture. Eye 2:1–11 1988

10 Rootman J. Frequency and differential diagnosis of orbital disease. In: Rootman J (ed) Diseases of the orbit. Philadelphia: Lippincott, 1988:131

11 Phelps C D, Thompson H S, Ossoinig K C. The diagnosis and prognosis of atypical carotid-cavernous fistula (red-eyed shunt syndrome). Am J Ophthalmol 93:423–436 1982

12 MacNeill J R. Standardized echography in C. C. fistula. In: Ossoinig K C (ed) Ophthalmic echography. Dordrecht: Junk, 1987:521

13 Flaharty P M, Lieb W E, Sergott R C et al. Colour Doppler imaging: a new non-invasive technique to diagnose and monitor carotid cavernous fistulas. Arch Ophthalmol 109:522–526 1991

14 Kotval P S, Weitzner I, Tenner M S. Diagnosis of carotid-cavernous fistula by periorbital color Doppler imaging and pulsed Doppler volume flow analysis. J Ultrasound Med 9:101–106 1990

15 Atta H R. Standardized echography in a case of orbital varix. In: Till P (ed) Ophthalmic Echography, 13. Dordrecht: Kluwer, 1993:199–203

16 Ossoinig K C. Echographic differentiation of vascular tumours in the orbit. Docum Ophthalmol Proc Series 29:283–291 1981

17 Shields J A. Diagnosis and management of orbital tumours. Philadelphia: Saunders, 1989

18 Henderson J W. Orbital tumours. 2nd ed. New York: Stratton-Thieme, 1980:497

19 Rootman J. Inflammatory diseases. In: Rootman J (ed) Diseases of the orbit. Philadelphia: Lippincott, 1988:159

20 Hasenfratz G, Ossoinig K C. The diagnosis of orbital mucoceles and pyoceles with standardized echography. In: Hillman J S, Lemay M M (eds) Ophthalmic ultrasonography. Dordrecht: Junk, 1983:407

21 Coleman D J, Jack R L, Franzen L A. B-scan ultrasonography of orbital mucoceles. Eye Ear Nose Throat Mon 51:207 1972

9

Indications: orbit

Standardized echography is a valuable modality in the investigation of orbital disease.[1-8] Its merits, compared to computed tomographic (CT) scanning and magnetic resonance imaging (MRI), lie in its inherent low cost and safety. In experienced hands, standardized echography is capable of supplying numerous acoustic data, particularly 'kinetic' and 'quantitative' information which aids in the tissue differentiation of lesions.[1,9] In addition, it is more sensitive in the detection of subtle orbital abnormalities such as engorgement of orbital veins,[10] mild thickening of extraocular muscles[11] and distension of the optic nerve sheaths.[12] Associated ocular abnormalities such as disc oedema, chorioretinal thickening and detachment, and indentation of the globe are all better identified on ultrasonography.

CT and MRI scans, on the other hand, are superior to echography in the 'topographic' depiction of anatomical features and in displaying the orbital apex, bony walls, adjacent intracranial compartment, and air sinuses. They also provide a permanent pictorial record, which may be used as a reference during orbital surgery.

In practice, echography is employed as a rapid initial investigation, which alone may confirm the clinical diagnosis, and acts as a screening test, pointing out the need for further expensive and invasive investigations. It also complements other tests by demonstrating the often subtle orbital soft-tissue abnormalities associated with a bony defect and intracranial lesions such as arterio-venous fistulae and superior orbital fissure/sphenoid wing masses.

In this chapter the echographic evaluation of orbital diseases is illustrated within the clinical context. Many of the echographic findings have already been described in Chapters 7 and 8.

Orbital echography is indicated in the following:

- Proptosis and globe displacement.
- Abnormal lid positions and oedema.
- Some cases of motility disturbance.
- Some cases of ocular/orbital pain.

- Uniocular injection and rise in intraocular pressure.
- Some cases of optic disc oedema/atrophy and vascular retinal occlusion.
- Choroidal folds.
- Orbital trauma.

PROPTOSIS AND ABNORMAL LID POSITIONS

Before embarking on a detailed examination, the echographer needs to exclude 'pseudo-exophthalmos' as a cause of proptosis. This is commonly encountered in cases of congenital high myopia and posterior staphyloma, where the axial eye length is exceedingly long (Figure 9.1). Pseudo-exophthalmos is ruled out by measuring the axial eye length on A-scan and observing the globe contour on B-scan.

If true proptosis is present the examiner proceeds with the scanning. As thyroid eye disease is the most common cause of proptosis, evaluating the extraocular muscles seems to be the next logical step. Muscle measurements are performed with A-scan as previously described. It is important to conduct the examination in the primary position of gaze, to prevent contraction and relaxation of muscles. Whilst the patient's eye is positioned at the primary gaze, the examiner proceeds to measure the optic nerve width, and, if it is enlarged, to perform the 30° test (see Chapter 7). A B-scan is then carried out to confirm the A-scan findings.

If the extraocular muscles and optic nerve are normal and symmetrical between the two orbits, B-scan is further utilized to screen the orbital fat for mass lesion and enlarged orbital vein, and to illustrate irregularities in the bone line and adjacent sinuses. If these are found, further examination with standardized A-scan, and in some cases Doppler ultrasound, is performed to

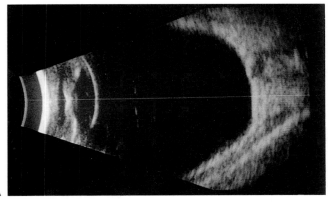

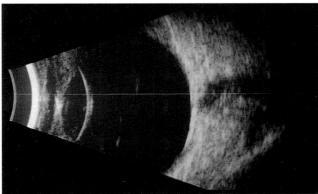

A   B

Figure 9.1 Axial myopia/posterior staphyloma causing 'pseudo-exophthalmos'. Figure 9.1A shows an abnormal ectatic posterior globe wall and long axial length, as compared to the normal eye in Figure 9.1B

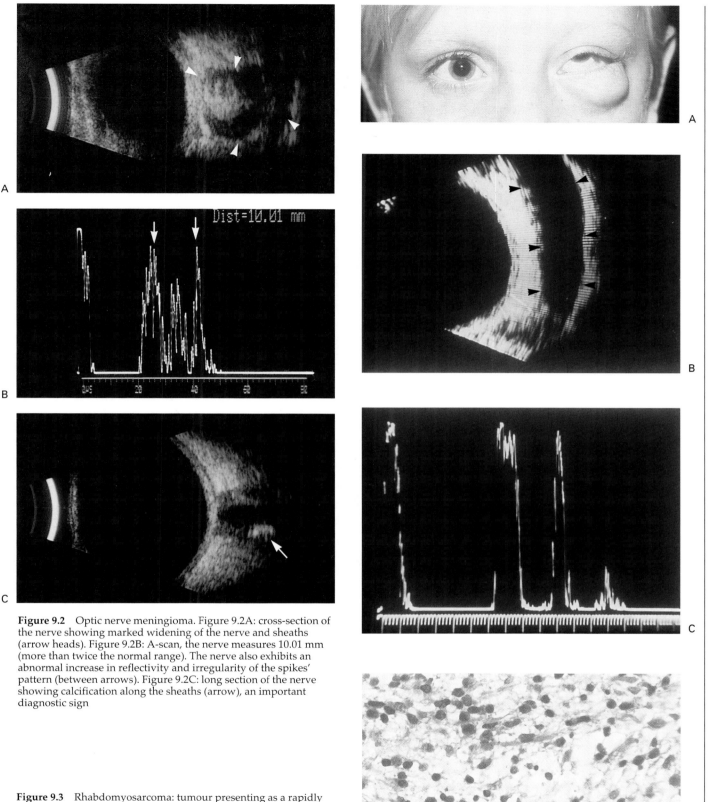

Figure 9.2 Optic nerve meningioma. Figure 9.2A: cross-section of the nerve showing marked widening of the nerve and sheaths (arrow heads). Figure 9.2B: A-scan, the nerve measures 10.01 mm (more than twice the normal range). The nerve also exhibits an abnormal increase in reflectivity and irregularity of the spikes' pattern (between arrows). Figure 9.2C: long section of the nerve showing calcification along the sheaths (arrow), an important diagnostic sign

Figure 9.3 Rhabdomyosarcoma: tumour presenting as a rapidly expanding mass in the anterior inferior orbital compartment (Figure 9.3A), causing upward displacement of the globe. The B-scan (Figure 9.3B) shows a dark mass infiltrating the orbital floor (arrow heads). The A-scan (Figure 9.3C) demonstrates a low-reflective lesion. Low reflectivity is due to the small, homogeneous histological structure of such tumours (Figure 9.3D) (Courtesy of S F Byrne)

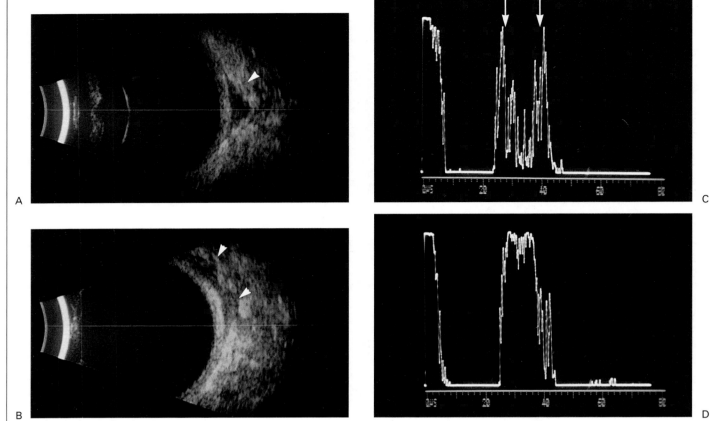

Figure 9.4 Metastatic orbital tumour from breast carcinoma. Figure 9.4A: a vertical macula. Figure 9.4B: a transverse-6P section showing infiltrative, poorly outlined pockets of tumour adjacent to the globe wall (arrow heads). Figure 9.4C: an A-scan of the tumour. The lesion is low-reflective and irregularly structured with the characteristic 'V' pattern commonly seen in orbital malignancy. Figure 9.4D: A-scan of the normal fellow orbit.

collect the maximum acoustic data and make a diagnosis.

Findings that are detected on echography will depend on the age of the patient and the presenting clinical features. In adults, apart from thyroid orbitopathy, possible lesions include cavernous haemangioma, orbital vascular lesions, pseudotumours, and optic nerve meningioma (Figure 9.2). In children rhabdomyosarcoma should always be considered, particularly if proptosis is rapid and associated with acute orbital signs. These tumours may occur anywhere in the orbit and may be located very anteriorly, under the lid and conjunctival fornices. Paraocular and peripheral transocular scanning are therefore required to reveal such tumours (Figure 9.3). Other lesions in children include capillary haemangioma, lymphangioma, dermoid cysts, and optic nerve glioma. In the elderly, lymphoma and carcinoma, often invading from neighbouring regions or from a distant metastasis, should be suspected (Figure 9.4). Other frequent causes include orbital mucoceles, cavernous haemangioma, and chronic dural sinus fistula. It is worth remembering that enophthalmos can be a manifestation of a scirrhous metastatic carcinoma, for example from the breast.

Lacrimal gland and fossa lesions produce upper-lid S-shaped swelling and mechanical ptosis (Figure 9.5). While the normal lacrimal gland is indistinguishable from the surrounding fat (Figure 7.22), swelling of the gland from oedema or venous congestion results in

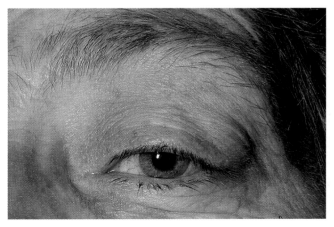

Figure 9.5 Lacrimal gland swelling, producing ptosis and an S-shaped upper lid displacement

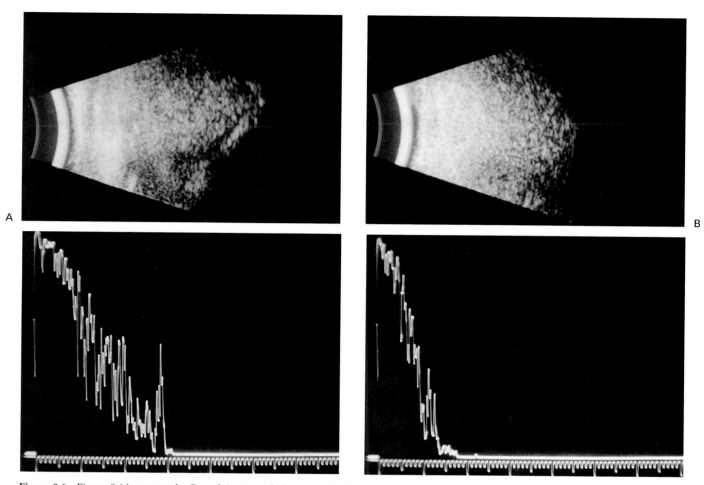

Figure 9.6 Figure 9.6A: paraocular B- and A-scans of a lacrimal gland enlarged as a result of oedema and venous congestion. Figure 9.6B: the same scans of opposite gland

widening of the fat pattern without alterations in the spikes' characteristics on A-scan (Figure 9.6). Infiltration of the lacrimal gland, however, produces a defect as well as a widening in the fat pattern. Within the defect, the spikes' features alter, becoming low-reflective and regular in inflammatory and lymphomatous infiltration (Figure 7.23) and irregular and more reflective in epithelial tumours of the gland such as benign mixed tumours (Figure 9.7). Examination of the bone of the lacrimal fossa may yield useful information, e.g. erosion from malignant tumour.

Considerable experience, however, is needed to be able to 'tissue differentiate' lacrimal gland lesions with echography, and other investigations are invariably required before the correct diagnosis is reached.[13]

OCULAR MOTILITY DISTURBANCES AND ORBITAL PAIN

Disturbance of ocular motility, especially when accompanied by pain, can result from ocular myositis, posterior scleritis, and, if there is significant proptosis, orbital pseudotumour. All of these lesions are considered variants of the same disease, and on echography present either alone or in combination. If the vision is affected, involvement of the optic nerve sheaths is suspected. Thyroid orbitopathy should again be ruled out as a cause of motility restriction.

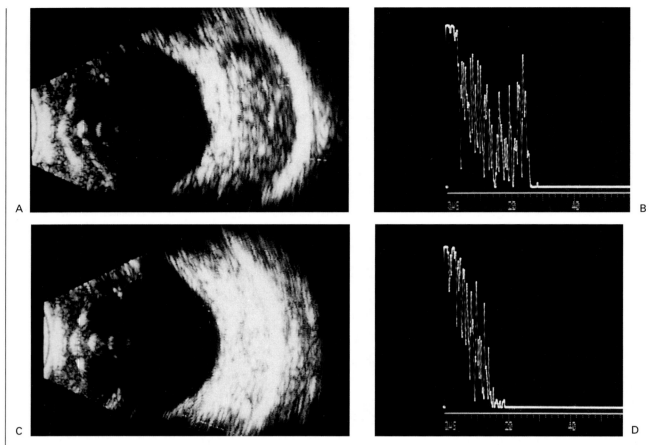

Figure 9.7 Figure 9.7A: B-scan. A large 'benign mixed tumour' of the lacrimal gland is seen indenting the globe. Figure 9.7B: A-scan showing widening and irregularity of the echo-pattern. Figures 9.7C and 9.7D: scans of the normal gland

Severe ophthalmoplegia accompanied by ocular pain with or without proptosis is frequently caused by Tolosa Hunt syndrome, orbital apex lesion, or cavernous sinus lesion. Echographic features of orbital venous congestion are usually present in such conditions.

Painless ophthalmoplegia can result from granulo-matous or neoplastic infiltration of the extraocular muscles (Figure 9.8). Echography is therefore of value in ruling out these disorders.

Pain without other symptoms or signs of orbital disease invariably produces negative findings on echography.

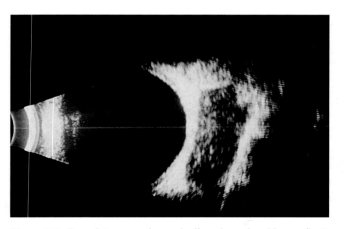

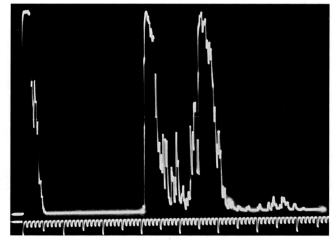

Figure 9.8 B- and A-scans of a markedly enlarged and low-reflective medial rectus muscle. The diagnosis proved to be a lymphomatous infiltration

UNIOCULAR INJECTION AND RISE IN INTRAOCULAR PRESSURE

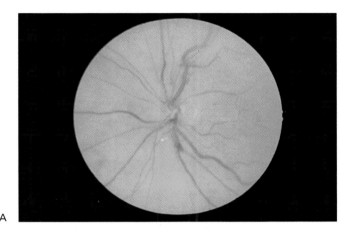

A

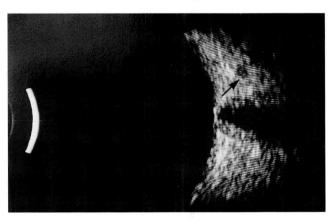

B

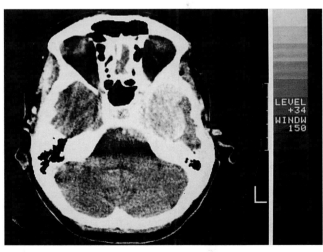

C

Figure 9.9 Patient presenting with a picture of left venous stasis retinopathy (Figure 9.9A). Echography (Figure 9.9B) demonstrated enlargement of the extraocular muscle, distension of the optic nerve, and engorgement of the orbital vein (arrow) on the same side. CT scan (Figure 9.9C) revealed a large meningioma, occupying most of the left middle cranial fossa

An interference with the orbital venous outflow should be suspected in cases of uniocular rise in intraocular pressure associated with injection and dilatation of conjunctival vessels. Disc oedema and retinal venous stasis may also be encountered. In such cases a degree of proptosis, limitation of ocular movements, and bruit may also be present.

These features are seen in a severe form in direct, fast-flow carotid-cavernous fistula, commonly caused by gunshot head injury or fracture of the base of the skull. Less marked features are encountered in slow-flow, dural sinus fistula.[10] This is a spontaneous lesion, which is more common in patients of middle to advanced age with no previous history of trauma. Obstruction of the venous outflow can also be caused by a mass lesion in the superior orbital fissure, orbital apex, or cavernous sinus region. Orbital venous congestion not caused by A-V fistula or a mass lesion may develop following thrombosis of the superior ophthalmic vein.

On echography, the extraocular muscles are uniformly swollen in one orbit, without alteration in their reflectivity. Congestion may occasionally be bilateral – e.g. in a large carotid-cavernous fistula – but is invariably asymmetrical. In addition to muscle enlargement, engorgement of orbital vein(s) is a constant feature. This is usually detected in the supra-nasal aspect of the orbit (Figures 8.9, 8.10). Widening of the fat pattern and, in severe cases, distension of the optic nerve sheaths and thickening and detachment of the chorioretinal layer may also develop. Doppler ultrasound is helpful in demonstrating an increase and 'arterialization' of blood flow in the orbit.

CT scan, MRI and/or cerebral angiography are called upon in such cases to isolate the underlying lesion. Figure 9.9 illustrates a case of orbital venous congestion due to a large meningioma in the middle cranial fossa.

OPTIC DISC ABNORMALITIES AND CENTRAL RETINAL VEIN OCCLUSION

Some orbital disease may produce disc oedema and abnormalities in the retinal circulation. In such cases, echography can play a role in their investigation. Optic disc swelling is verified on B-scan. Buried disc drusen are often difficult to detect clinically, but owing to their high calcium content they are easily demonstrated on echography (Figure 9.10), thus obviating the need for fluorescein angiography and radiological tests. Papilloedema due to increased intracranial pressure produces a strongly positive 30°

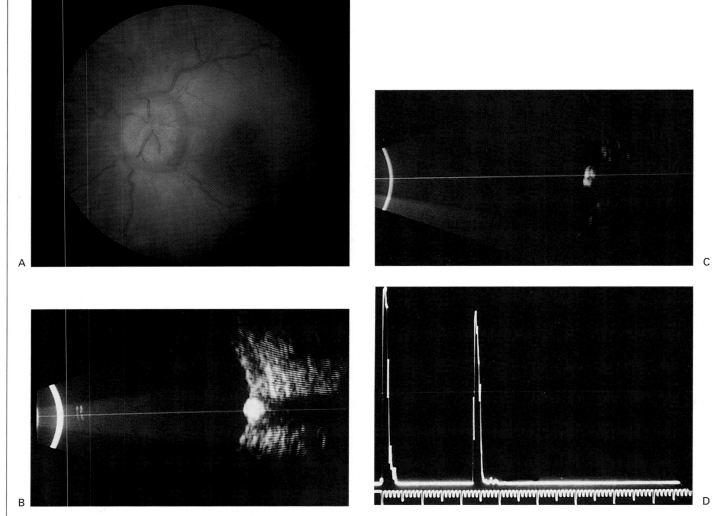

Figure 9.10 Buried optic disc drüsen. Figure 9.10A: disc appearance on presentation. Figure 9.10B: medium-gain B-scan showing a high-reflective round opacity at the optic nerve head, giving rise to shadowing. Figures 9.10C and 9.10D: low-reflective B- and A-scans. Only the drusen remains reflective owing to its high calcium content

test, indicating fluid distension of the optic nerve sheaths (Figure 9.11). Echography is helpful in the diagnosis of pseudotumour cerebri and in the management of cases requiring optic nerve fenestration.

Optic disc atrophy can result from a compressive optic nerve or an adjacent orbital mass lesion. Abnormal optico-ciliary shunt vessel may be associated with optic nerve meningioma. Venous stasis retinopathy, especially if associated with other orbital signs, should be investigated with echography to exclude obstruction of the orbital venous outflow, as described above.

CHOROIDAL FOLDS

Choroidal folds should be distinguished from retinal striae. The latter is an abnormality in the inner retinal surface or vitreo-retinal interface, and is commonly located at the macular area. Fluorescein angiography[14] and ultrasound examination[15,16] are two useful tests in the investigation of choroidal folds (Figure 9.12).

Choroidal folds may be 'idiopathic' where no ocular or orbital cause is found.[15] In such cases, a history of progressive hypermetropia is usually obtained, and flattening of the posterior globe wall with corresponding reduction in the axial eye length is detected on echography. Thickening of the chorio-retinal layer is also encountered in some of these cases.

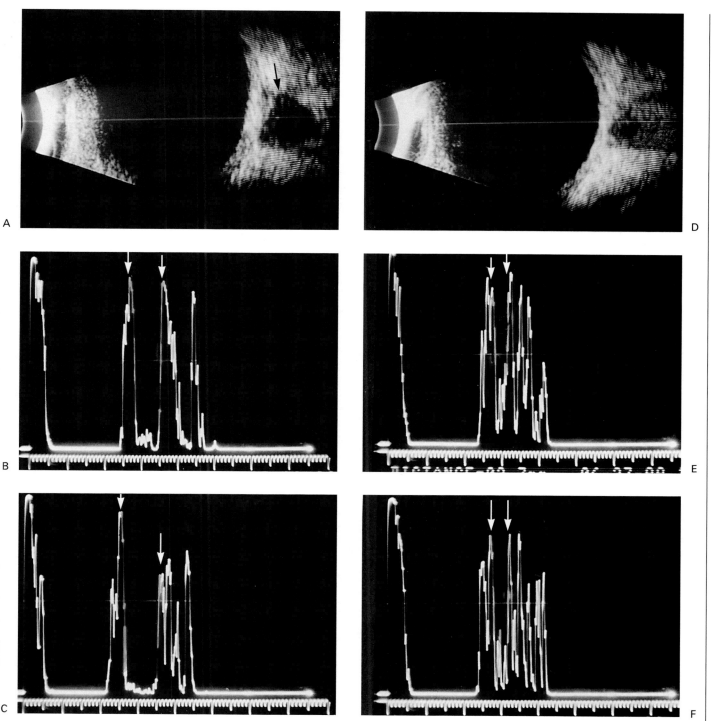

Figure 9.11 Pseudotumour cerebri. Figure 9.11A: a transverse B-scan of the optic nerve at primary position of gaze. Figures 9.11B and 9.11C: A-scans of the anterior and posterior segment of the nerve at primary position. Note the marked widening of the nerve. Figures 9.11D, 9.11E, and 9.11F: the same sections after 30° abduction. Significant reduction of nerve diameter is noted (arrows), indicating distension of nerve sheaths

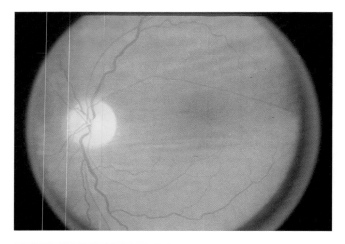

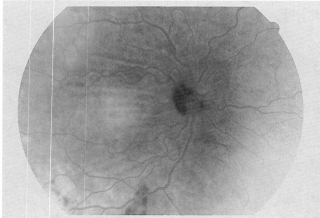

Figure 9.12 Colour photograph and fluorescein angiogram of choroidal folds – an important indication for echography

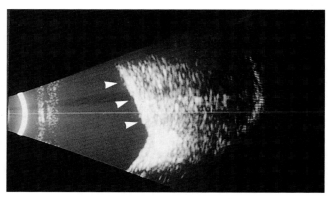

Figure 9.13 Choroidal folds may result from indentation of the globe by a retrobulbar mass, such as the one seen in this example of intra-conal cavernous haemangioma (arrow heads)

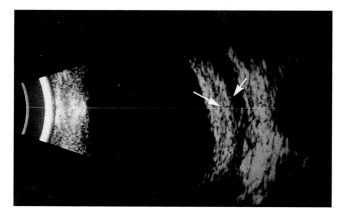

Figure 9.14 Marked thickening of the globe wall (left arrow) and episcleral space (right arrow) in posterior scleritis presenting clinically with choroidal folds

Orbital causes of choroidal folds include large retrobulbar optic nerve swelling, intra-conal mass lesion e.g. cavernous haemangioma, severe thyroid orbitopathy, large lacrimal gland lesion, and orbital haemorrhage and cellulitis. Indentation of the globe being a common denominator in these cases (Figure 9.13). Posterior scleritis is also a frequent cause of choroidal folds (9.14).

ORBITAL TRAUMA

Echography plays a role in the evaluation of orbital trauma. Abnormalities that could be demonstrated include blow-out fracture (Figure 9.15), orbital haemorrhage and emphysema (Figure 9.16), and avulsion of the optic nerve (Figure 9.17).

Echography is also useful in the detection of concomitant intraocular injuries, particularly if fundoscopy is hampered by lid swelling and media opacities. In cases of intraocular foreign bodies, echography is of value in establishing whether the foreign body has penetrated into the orbit (Figure 9.18). Owing to the high reflectivity and strong sound absorption property of the orbital fat, small foreign bodies lodged deep in the orbit may be missed on echography. Large foreign bodies, however, produce shadowing and are usually surrounded by (low-reflective) haemorrhage, making them easier to detect.

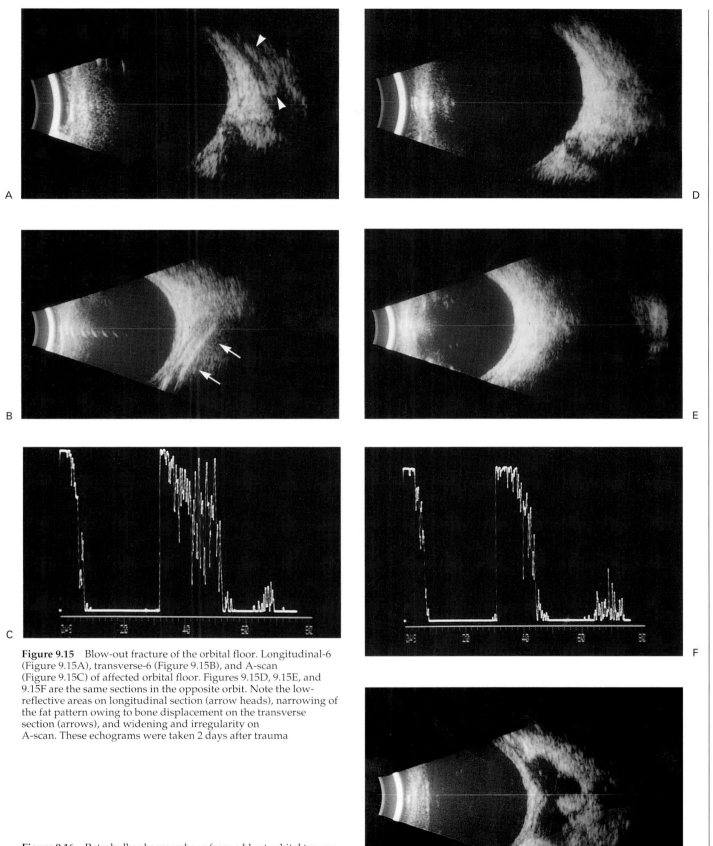

Figure 9.15 Blow-out fracture of the orbital floor. Longitudinal-6 (Figure 9.15A), transverse-6 (Figure 9.15B), and A-scan (Figure 9.15C) of affected orbital floor. Figures 9.15D, 9.15E, and 9.15F are the same sections in the opposite orbit. Note the low-reflective areas on longitudinal section (arrow heads), narrowing of the fat pattern owing to bone displacement on the transverse section (arrows), and widening and irregularity on A-scan. These echograms were taken 2 days after trauma

Figure 9.16 Retrobulbar haemorrhage from a blunt orbital trauma, appearing as an irregularly outlined dark area behind the globe. Follow-up echography after 2 weeks showed complete resolution of the haemorrhage

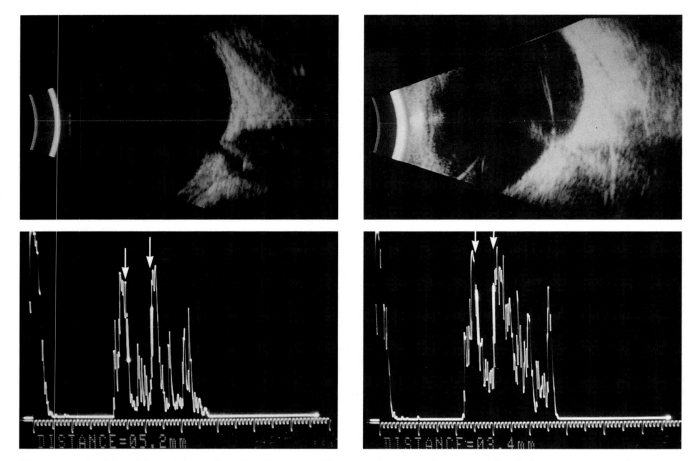

Figure 9.17 Avulsion of the optic nerve. Left: B- and A-scans of the nerve taken soon after trauma. Note the large excavation at the nerve head, and widening of the nerve diameter, which measures 5.2 mm on A-scan. Right: scans taken 12 weeks after injury. The 'gap' at the nerve head has been closed, probably with gliosis, attaching it to a thick V-shaped posterior vitreous detachment. The nerve diameter on A-scan now measures 3.4 mm, a reduction presumably due to absorption of subarachnoid haemorrhage within the nerve sheaths

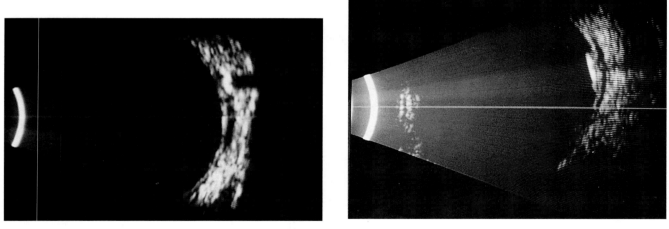

Figure 9.18 Intraorbital foreign body. Figure 9.18A: a small foreign body (FB), giving rise to shadowing, is seen in the immediate retrobulbar area; this is compared with a FB lying within the globe (Figure 9.18B)

REFERENCES

1 Byrne S F, Glaser J S. Orbital tissue differentiation with standardized echography. Ophthalmology 90:1071–1090 1983

2 Hodes B L, Weinberg P. A combined approach for the diagnosis of orbital disease. Arch Ophthalmol 95:781–788 1977

3 Ossoinig K C, Till P. Ten years study on clinical echography in orbital disease. Bibl Ophthalmol 83:200–216 1975

4 Ossoinig K C. The role of clinical echography in modern diagnosis of periorbital and orbital lesions. In: Orbital Centre of the Amsterdam University Eye Hospital (ed) Proceedings of the 3rd International Symposium on Orbital Disorders. The Hague: Junk, 1978:496–540

5 Byrne S F. Standardized echography in the differentiation of orbital lesions. Surv Ophthalmol 29:226–228 1984

6 Hasenfratz G, Lewan U. Results of standardized echography in orbital diseases. A review of 311 cases. In: Till P (ed) Ophthalmic echography, 13. Dordrecht: Kluwer, 1993:135–144

7 Harrie R P. Standardized echography of the orbit (review). Doc Ophthalmol Pro Series 48:445–451 1987

8 Till P, Hauff W. Differential diagnosis results of clinical echography in orbital tumors. Doc Ophthalmol Pro Series 29:277–282 1981

9 Byrne S F. Standardized echography of the eye and orbit. Neuroradiology 28:618–640 1986

10 Phelps C D, Thompson H S, Ossoinig K C. The diagnosis and prognosis of atypical carotid-cavernous fistula (red-eyed shunt syndrome). Am J Ophthalmol 93:423–436 1982

11 Dick A D, Nangia V, Atta H. Standardised echography in the differential diagnosis of extraocular muscle enlargement. Eye 6:610–617 1992

12 Atta H R. Imaging of the optic nerve with standardised echography. Eye 2:358–366 1988

13 Balchunas W R, Quencer R M, Byrne S F. Lacrimal gland and fossa masses: evaluation by computed tomography and A-mode echography. Radiology 149:751–758 1983

14 Norton E W D. A characteristic fluorescein angiographic pattern in choroidal folds. Proc R Soc Med 62:119–128 1969

15 Atta H R, Byrne S F. The findings of standardized echography for choroidal folds. Arch Ophthalmol 106:1234–1241 1988

16 Cappaert W E, Purnell E W, Frank K E. Use of B-sector scan ultrasound in the diagnosis of benign choroidal folds. Am J Ophthalmol 84:375–379 1977

Glossary

A-scan: 'A' for amplitude. One-dimensional display of returning echoes, appearing as positive waves (spikes) from a baseline.

After-movements: The undulations of membranous opacities immediately after the cessation of eye movements.

Amplification, sound: Returning echoes need to be amplified in order that they may be detected and displayed on the screen. Amplification may be linear (high sensitivity and small dynamic range), logarithmic (low sensitivity and high dynamic range) or S-shaped (adequate sensitivity and dynamic range). The latter is an essential component in 'standardized' A-scan.

Amplitude: Height of spikes on A-scan. The higher the amplitude the stronger the returning echo.

Angle kappa: The angle of decline of the spikes' height on A-scan as the sound energy is attenuated along the beam path.

Artefact: Acoustic artefacts may be produced by (unwanted) external factors such as air bubbles trapped in the probe or poor contact between the globe and transducer. Internal or 'tissue' artefacts may aid the diagnosis, e. g. shadowing from calcium or a foreign body, and reverberation from a gun pellet.

Attenuation, sound: The reduction in intensity of returning echoes as the sound travels through media. This is caused by absorption, scatter, reflection, and refraction of sound waves.

Biometry: In vivo ultrasonic measurement of distances and diameters of tissues.

B-scan: 'B' for brightness. Two-dimensional display of returning echoes, appearing as dots of various brightness, depending on the intensity of the echo-sources.

Decibel scale (dB): A logarithmic scale used to express ratios of intensities and powers. It allows the conversion of large measurements into more practical, small numbers. Levels of sound gain and attenuation are expressed in this way.

Dynamic range: A function of sound amplification in A-scan; it describes in decibels the range of the spikes' amplitudes, from the weakest (5%) to the strongest (95%).

Gain: The function by which the amplitude of the display signal is changed. This can be achieved by altering the power of the transmitted pulse or the degree of amplification of returning echoes.

Grey scale: The ability on B-scan to display dots in numerous shades of grey, depending on the intensity of the echo-source.

Interface: The demarcation line between two media of different sound velocities.

Internal structure: The regularity in amplitude and spacing of spikes within tissues on A-scan. It correlates well with the regularity of histological structure.

Kinetic echography: The unique ultrasound capacity for evaluation of the mobility of tissues during performance of the examination – a feature not currently available in other imaging techniques.

Pachymetry: Ultrasonic measurement of corneal thickness.

Piezoelectric phenomenon: The ability of an element to transform an electric current into a mechanical, sound-emitting energy and vice versa. Piezoelectric crystals are normally housed at the tip of an ultrasound probe (transducer).

Quantitative echography: The A-scan analyses of spikes' height (reflectivity), internal structure, and sound attenuation, which are used to differentiate types of tissues.

Real-time scanning: The B-scan feature of displaying tissue movement as it occurs during examination. This is achieved by increasing the 'frame rate' to equal or exceed that of tissue movement.

Reflectivity: The intensity of echo-sources. On A-scan it is assessed by measuring the amplitude of spikes, and on B-scan by the brightness of the dots.

Resolution: The ability to distinguish two targets, placed close together, as two separate echo-sources. Resolution can be axial when targets are placed along the beam path, or lateral when they are lying 'across' the beam path.

Reverberations: Artefacts created by highly reflective interfaces, commonly produced by intraocular lenses and foreign bodies, particularly gun pellets. They appear as regularly spaced spikes on A-scan and concentric, curved lines on B-scan; both decrease in intensity along the beam path.

Shadowing: Strongly reflecting interfaces tend to prevent further propagation of sound energy, resulting in the 'shadowing' of more distal targets lying along the beam path. This is produced by air, calcification, and intraocular foreign bodies.

Tissue (T)-sensitivity: A specific sound gain, expressed in decibels (dB), employed in standardized A-scan examination. It is unique for each probe/instrument and is calibrated by using a 'tissue model'.

Topographic echography: The evaluation of shape (configuration), location, and borders (extension) of lesions in the eye and orbit.

Vector A-scan: A linear (amplitude) sampling of a portion of the B-scan. It provides a quick reference on reflectivity and distances (diameters). It should not be confused with 'standardized' A-scan.

Index